AUTISM LITE

LEADING OUR CHILD OFF THE SPECTRUM

KATHRYN TUCKER

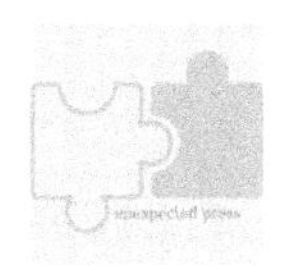

Copyright © 2020 by Unexpected Press

All rights reserved.

No part of this book may be reproduced in any form or by any electronic or mechanical means, including information storage and retrieval systems, without written permission from the author, except for the use of brief quotations in a book review.

This book is not intended to diagnose or as a substitute for the medical advice of physicians. The reader should consult with medical professionals for diagnoses and appropriate therapies and interventions.

The author has written under a pseudonym to protect her children's privacy. Most names in the book are also pseudonyms.

ISBN: 978-1-7359044-1-2

Library of Congress Control Number: 2020919405

To My Four—
I hope you will always come together to support and love each other the way you did for your sister when she needed you most.

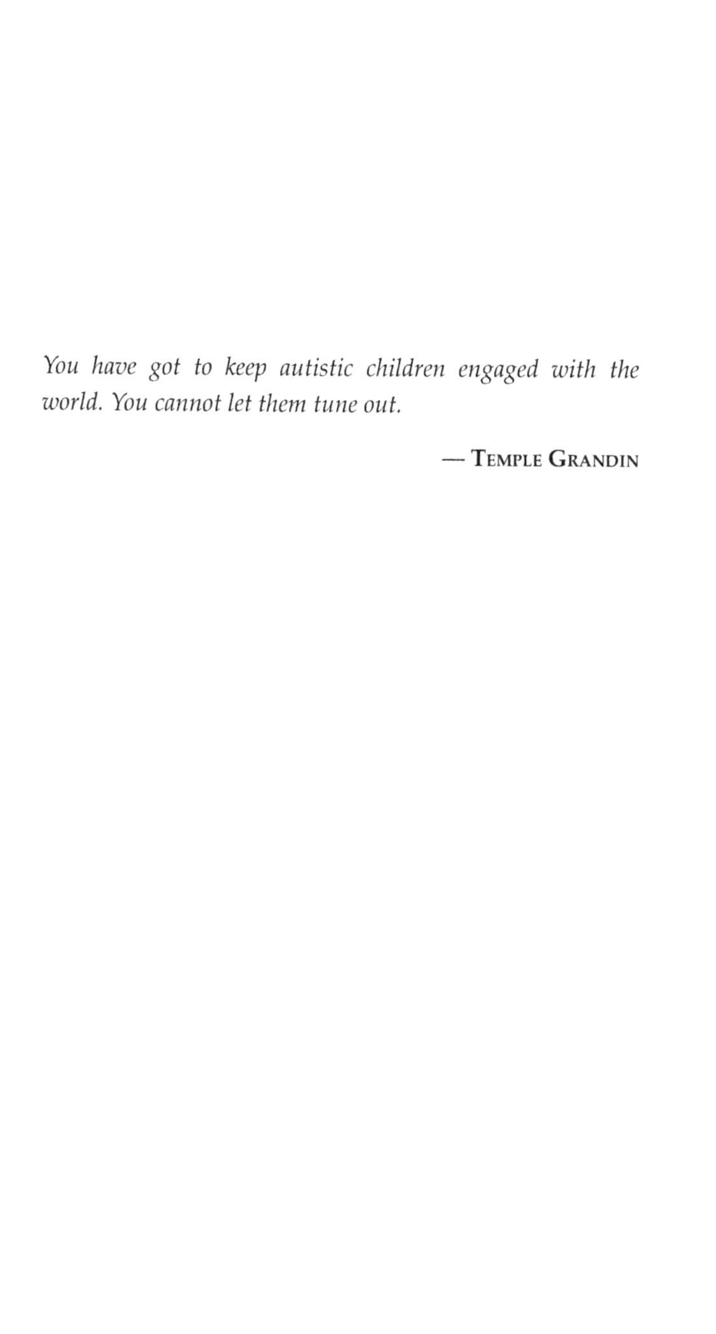

You have got to keep autistic children engaged with the world. You cannot let them tune out.

— Temple Grandin

CONTENTS

INTRODUCTION

Not Otherwise Specified

Autism is like a mysterious, invasive tree that grows differently inside each child on the spectrum. Some branches may be small and easy to snap off, while others grow thick and wild. The autism tree can hide itself well in young children. It seems almost dormant the first year or two, barely showing glimpses of its presence. When a few branches do start poking out into the open, they are often too subtle to hint at the greater tree within—and the earlier that tree is found, the easier to chop away at those branches forming a wall between the child and the outside world.

Two years ago, we discovered the autism tree manifesting in our daughter, Janie. Though we will never completely uproot that tree, Janie's story is a success story. No vaccine or pill can cure autism, but therapy—especially the therapies available today for this generation of children—can be incredibly effective at diminishing the disorder.

I felt blindsided the day our pediatrician first suggested that Janie might have autism. She was a playful two-year-old with a bold personality and symptoms so easy to miss, I had little idea that she struggled to communicate and socialize.

Nor did I realize how quickly our family's lives would change. Everyone's focus would turn to Janie and how we could help her.

Janie was diagnosed with Pervasive Developmental Disorder Not Otherwise Specified (PDD-NOS), also known as mild autism. The "not otherwise specified" part of the diagnosis puzzled me, but also seemed apt since I could not specify myself exactly why and how she fit on the spectrum. I have never heard autism referred to as a nebulous condition, but I found it so, initially. Only several months later did I truly wrap my head around her diagnosis.

Difficult to recognize in young children, mild autism too often flies under the radar. Janie's speech delay, her ability to play on her own for long periods, and her lack of interest in kids her age were noticeable, but not alarming to me at the time. Yet all of these indicators pointed to a child who does not understand communication or social situations—a child with autism. While we never expected one of our children to have special needs, we were extremely fortunate that our pediatrician picked up on Janie's autism at two years old.

Janie's progress has been nothing short of extraordinary because she has the capacity for it, but also because of the excellent therapists and teachers that helped her overcome many of her tendencies of autism. *Intensive therapy—the earlier the better—offers the best chance of preventing symptoms of autism from hardwiring for a child's lifetime.*

After the diagnosis, we dove deep into therapy. Early Intervention paired Janie with a psychologist named Megan, who practices a therapy for children with autism called the Early Start Denver Model (ESDM). This behavioral and developmental therapy teaches a specific set of skills through play and daily routine activities to build a child's relationships and develop social-emotional, cognitive, and language skills, fine and gross motor skills, and self-help skills.[1]

Megan worked with Janie several hours each week systematically identifying, reducing, and sometimes eradicating entirely many of her symptoms of autism. She trained our entire family to interact and play with Janie in ways that advanced her social and communication skills, so that we too became her therapists. The skills not intrinsic to Janie and not developing naturally, she learned through ESDM therapy with Megan and by extension, our family.

Megan became my conduit to Janie, explaining what I had not understood about my daughter and how differently she perceived the world. We have come to discover that Janie's mind is quite amazing and to cherish the parts of autism that make Janie, Janie, while also cutting back those branches of autism that isolate her. Megan drew Janie out of her inner world and into the world around her. If Megan ever needs a kidney, I will be the first in line.

The past two years have taken our family down an unexpected path—a path both challenging and fascinating. I write about Janie's autism partly for myself; writing is cathartic. It also helps me continue to better understand autism and Janie. While I am no expert on autism, I am now an expert on my daughter, her autism, and how to lessen or eliminate her symptoms.

I do not presume to know the best therapy for autism. Many therapies work, and which works best depends on the child. And I would never compare our experiences to that of a family with a child who has severe autism.

My daughter's autism was both a shock and an enigma to me. Raising general awareness of mild autism is crucial to identifying children on the spectrum and getting them the therapy they need from an early age. I hope that sharing Janie's story and the learning curve our family has traveled will be helpful and relatable to anyone with a child in their immediate or extended family, neighborhood, classroom, community group, or practice with mild autism—whether labeled PDD-NOS, Autism Spectrum Disorder (Level 1 or 2), high-functioning autism, or in my simple terms, autism lite.

PART I

DISAPPEARING CHILD

1

FINDING THE TREE

The Doctor's Appointment

Our pediatrician recognized the autism tree in Janie. It was mid-summer, and we were meeting Dr. Shaw for the first time at Janie's two-year checkup. With Janie on my lap reclining against my very pregnant belly, I tried to get comfortable in the polyester chair facing our new pediatrician and, unbeknownst to me at the time, a new reality for us. I never suspected the tree in my daughter.

I had been to dozens of well visits for my three kids, so expected a quick turnaround once the doctor walked in the room. But Dr. Shaw settled into her swivel stool and spent the first 20 minutes asking me questions about Janie, typing away at her laptop while I talked. She examined Janie, then sat down again to ask me more about two of my concerns: Janie seemed to recognize a variety of words, but rarely talked, and she had little interest in children her own age.

Dr. Shaw had also taken pause at what she called "social referencing"—Janie not looking to me for clarification in a new situation. When Dr. Shaw showed her an unfamiliar toy, Janie did not gauge my reaction. Her eye contact seemed fine to me. I did not understand the significance. I had yet to realize how little I understood about Janie.

Dr. Shaw suggested a developmental evaluation. When I asked her what that meant, she replied not unkindly, but directly, "Well, we would test Janie for developmental disorders, such as autism."

That gave me pause. So far I had really liked Dr. Shaw, but this comment came out of left field for me.

I had switched pediatricians a few times over the years trying to find the right fit for my kids and for me. Our first one set the bar high with her easy, yet thorough manner and thoughtful advice. After she moved, I found the next two pediatricians arrogant and aloof. Our fourth was more friendly than knowledgeable. The fifth was gruff, but I stuck with her for three years until Janie had an allergic reaction to penicillin. The pediatrician attributed her swollen feet and hands to an airplane trip, and after a painful night for Janie in the emergency room, I was again in the market for a different doctor.

We could not schedule an appointment with our new pediatrician in time for Janie's two-year checkup, so we met with another doctor in the practice, who turned out to be Dr. Shaw, a developmental pediatrician with expertise in diagnosing behavioral and developmental disorders. Looking back, I had no idea how fortuitous Janie's penicillin allergy would turn out to be, setting in motion our meeting with Dr. Shaw. Many doctors would not have picked up on Janie's symptoms of autism, certainly not the last one.

I scrutinized Dr. Shaw as she spoke to me, her open and professional demeanor, her curly brown hair and wire-rimmed glasses, her belly just about as pregnant as mine. My feelings wavered, and I could not settle my opinion of her—and her suggestion that Janie might have autism.

"Let's definitely get going with Early Intervention to address the speech delay," Dr. Shaw said. "The evaluation is up to you, but I would recommend it."

Although developmental issues were Dr. Shaw's area of expertise, I assumed she was being overly thorough—Janie could not possibly have autism. Plus Dr. Shaw was young, in her late twenties or early thirties, pregnant with her first child, while I was on round four. I did not doubt her integrity or intelligence; I doubted the necessity of an evaluation.

Autism is a heavy word. I gave a vague commitment about setting up an evaluation and headed out with Janie, my head spinning.

About Us

Our family's story begins 14 years earlier and 3,000 miles away. Both originally east coasters, my husband Christopher and I met in San Francisco. I came west straight out of college and worked at public relations agencies before settling into a career in corporate communications at a technology company. Christopher landed in California after graduate school, taking a position in business development at an emerging Internet company.

Christopher was too much fun not to marry. He was almost always in a good mood, worked hard, and shared my values and sense of humor. We enjoyed our twenties on the west coast, but both wanted to be closer to family once we had children of our own. We moved to Boston a couple years after we married.

San Francisco is not an easy city to leave. While I longed for the beauty of northern California and being outdoors so much of the year, I fell in love with Boston too. The city's history feels almost palpable—from the worn brick sidewalks to the stunning architecture of Boston's churches and brownstones. Our careers took a new path as well. Christopher and I decided to start our own business and launched an Internet company together.

About a year and half after we moved to Boston, our first daughter, Sarah, arrived. She inherited my green eyes and brown hair, streaked with lighter shades of Christopher's strawberry blond. I stopped working soon after Sarah was born. I enjoyed being a full-time mom, notwithstanding the lack of sleep and sometime isolation of motherhood. We left city living for suburbia just before our son, Luke, was born two years later.

I did not realize Sarah was an easy baby until I had Luke. Sarah was calm, always observing everything around her. I often watched her taking it all in, wondering what she was thinking. Luke was colicky, seeming to only find comfort when held, which was exhausting. Once the colic and his near constant ear infections subsided, the pendulum swung the other way for him—he has been my most relaxed and easy-going child ever since. Luke's light brown baby hair turned pure blond in the summers by the time he was a toddler. He resembled Sarah so closely with their olive skin and fair hair that people often mistook them for twins.

Sarah's manner was careful, thoughtful, and quiet. Luke's was similar, although as soon as he started crawling, I could see the boy/girl genetics at play as he went straight for the electrical sockets. Luke followed Sarah like a puppy dog. Contrary to her gentle demeanor, for a time Sarah rarely walked by Luke without knocking him over. His loyalty did pay off—they eventually became close playmates. They still get along unusually well for siblings.

When Sarah was three years old and Luke one, our dotcom bubble burst. The next few years were shadowed by financial hardships that took a toll on Christopher and me. We came out the other end, but the happy-go-lucky attitudes of our younger selves were altered. We changed in other ways too, learning to appreciate more deeply and taking very little for granted.

Sarah continued to be pensive and mature for her age. At five-years-old, she was the first person I told when I found out I was pregnant again. Luke developed into a lighthearted and curious little boy, often asking me funny questions, once if I had any monkey's phone numbers. When I told Luke about my pregnancy, he made clear he preferred a brother. He later figured that siblings must go in a pattern, so was unsurprised and resigned to the news when I called from the hospital to tell the kids they had a new sister. According to my in-laws, Sarah ran in circles celebrating.

Janie was petite in every way with soft, light brown hair and green eyes like her siblings. She and I both had low temperatures just after her birth, so the nurses put her tiny body on my chest and covered us in a heated blanket. I savored those moments warming up to each other.

The next month, Christopher accepted a position at an Internet company that put us back on a secure path financially. Sarah and Luke were old enough by then (six and four respectively) to help out with their new sister, delivering pacifiers and bottles, and even changing diapers once in a while.

Janie was a healthy baby and quick to smile. While she enjoyed the attention of her brother and sister, she was also content on her own, more so than Sarah and Luke had been. All of Janie's milestones came later than with her siblings—sitting up, crawling, walking. Even her teeth took unusually long to break through. Her delayed speech did not seem too out of the ordinary to me. I thought her personality more introverted, like her sister.

Janie grew into a happy and affectionate toddler, a disposition that belied her disorder. She laughed often, snuggled anyone nearby, and engaged readily with her brother and sister, although rarely with children her own age.

The summer Janie turned two, Christopher and I were in our late thirties and had just bought a house in a coastal New England town. It was in a new development going up on a cul-de-sac off a busy street. Our only real stress that summer was my pregnancy. My body was rebelling against its upcoming fourth cesarean section, and the baby faced several risks. We were worried about the baby, but overall in a good place the day I took Janie to the doctor for her two-year checkup.

That day autism became a part of our family.

2

CLUES FROM TODDLERHOOD

Janie's First Early Intervention Evaluation

Janie did not walk and barely talked by the time she was 15 months old. She spoke just two words: "yeah" and "go." She answered "yeah" to most questions, so there was no understanding behind the word. She stopped answering questions altogether a few months later. She did babble and said "mama" and "dada," but never in reference to Christopher or me.

To our previous pediatrician's credit, she had recommended an Early Intervention (EI) assessment at Janie's 15-month well visit. EI provides therapeutic services for children from birth to age three with developmental delays or disabilities.[1] EI services are available across the country and covered by the state and insurance. Parents incur very little cost. Therapists work with children in their home or daycare. EI, to me, is an almost magical organization, easy to deal with and tremendously helpful on every level.

The lovely team of women from our local EI chapter rolled into our townhouse on a sunny fall day with toys for Janie and documents for me. Our EI supervisor, Ann Marie, sat down with me and asked all about Janie, who had just started walking the week before. The developmental therapist and physical therapist settled on the floor presenting toys to Janie in such a warm and subdued manner that she was climbing all over them within a few minutes. Another specialist who took notes rounded out the team.

At the time, Janie cozied up to just about anyone. Number three on the totem pole, she was a bit starved for attention. I remember many mornings scrambling to get Sarah and Luke fed and ready for school in time while Janie fussed in her exersaucer, reaching her arms towards me to be picked up. I never left her there long, but long enough that she learned to entertain herself. She scraped out her afternoon naps in the car during school pick-ups. She tagged along to her siblings' activities more often than her own. So when a new person showed up, Janie was quite friendly and interactive. She had very little separation anxiety. This all changed over the next several months.

The EI team tested Janie in five areas: adaptive skills (feeding, dressing, hygiene, independence, and safety awareness), personal-social skills (interaction with adults and peers, self-awareness, and social development), communication skills (understanding and communicating with gestures and words), motor skills (movement and coordination), and cognitive skills (how a child explores and interacts with their environment, such as attention, problem solving, and discrimination skills).

Janie brought a ball over to the physical therapist, and they took turns rolling it back and forth. The therapists hid toys under a tiny blanket to see if she could find them, stacked blocks, looked at books, and nested cups with Janie. They eventually moved over to her high chair for more testing with Cheerios, crayons, and paper. Janie smiled and clapped when praised, and pointed at pictures in books to hear their labels, engaging the therapists with eye contact and joint attention (conscious sharing of interest in something by two people). During the activities, she showed positive and negative emotions, followed some directions, imitated speech, and babbled.

In her report, Ann Marie noted, "Janie is a good communicator, using eye contact, gestures, and joint attention well to socialize with others and get her needs met. She has just a few words at this time. Although very engaged socially, Janie did not identify familiar people or objects when named."

Ann Marie asked me if Janie could point to different parts of the body. While I had quizzed Sarah and Luke regularly as toddlers on body parts, I could not recall ever asking Janie. Could she follow a simple direction, like "Get the ball"? I rarely gave her directions.

I was somewhat mortified by my apparent laziness with Janie. Granted, I had less one-on-one time with her than I'd had with my older two. My parenting books were by then collecting dust, and maybe I relied too much on the assumption she would learn by osmosis from her siblings.

After an hour and half of testing, the EI team talked amongst themselves quietly, took notes, and then told me their findings. In our state, a score of 77 or below in one or more areas qualifies a child for EI services (average scores lie between 85–115). In the case of a "clinical judgment," EI may offer services to a child who does not fall below that score if the therapists believe an area of delay needs to be addressed. Janie did not qualify in any area; every score fell in the average range. All in all, they found her very social and communicative, even without words.

Ann Marie wrote in her assessment, "It is unclear at this time how much Janie understands as she is not yet following directions or looking to people when named. No other developmental concerns are noted."

They did not suspect autism. They had very little reason to, at the time. Her symptoms became more pronounced over the coming months.

I copied down all of their suggestions. They told me that Janie would focus more on walking and physical development than talking for the next few months, but if I did not see a big jump in her speech by 21 months, I should have her evaluated again. Although they could not have said it more gently, when they recommended I "engage more with Janie," it stung. And then they left with their smiles and toys—and good advice in their wake.

Quiet Janie

I took Janie shopping with me for a few hours one day soon after the EI evaluation. I joked afterwards, with some concern, that she felt more like a purse than a child. From car seat to stroller to stores and back again, she did not make a peep. I had one-sided conversations with Janie all day long, asking her questions, commenting on things we saw, singing songs she loved—but stopped waiting for a response since I never got one. Sarah and Luke are naturally reserved like me, so I thought Janie simply had the same temperament.

When Janie did start making some noise, it was to sing rather than talk. I signed us up for a music class together shortly after she turned one. Janie sat on my lap like a little monk, silently observing. Sarah had been exactly the same as a toddler, with focused eyes and a passive expression in new situations. When kids swarmed around a basket of toys at gym class, Sarah hung back until the seas parted. Only after she was comfortable and understood a new experience would she participate.

When Sarah started preschool at age three, she cried every day for the first six weeks, often from start to finish. She asked when her mommy was coming so often that the other kids in the class would all yell, "After the good-bye song!" I worried the preschool director would kick her out of the program, but she eventually warmed up and thrived.

So I likened Janie's reaction to new situations to Sarah's at her age, as they were similar—to a degree. They both needed time to sort out the world around them, but once Sarah got the lay of the land, she could move on. Without the communication and social skills intuitive to most children, Janie sometimes never got the lay of the land. To make sense of things and in a way, I think, to cope, Janie memorized.

In several months of music classes Janie often smiled, but had barely made a sound. She stayed planted in my lap when the teacher sprinkled tiny instruments all over the rug, and the other toddlers scrambled for drums, clackers, and shakers. She pulled on me to carry her when everyone danced around the circle.

The day Janie finally broke her silence she was about 20 months old. The teacher was singing a song that Janie had heard many times in class. In the middle of the song, she softly started singing along. Stunned to hear her voice, everyone stopped singing for a moment. I realized soon after that when Janie listened to music, sometimes staring at the static iTunes screen on my computer, she was actually hard at work. Memorizing was her tool to help understand what was not coming to her naturally.

Janie also memorized her books. I read to her a few times a day, and she would continue to look at books for long periods by herself. One afternoon when I finished reading Sandra Boynton's *Oh My, Oh My, Oh Dinosaurs* to her, she picked it up and recited the entire book back to me hardly missing a word, even imitating my tone of voice. I watched her on the video monitor at naptime while she paged through books telling the story as if reading it aloud.

Janie could repeat words, but had no idea how to use words to communicate. When I asked her to identify pictures in books, such as "Find the horse," she could find it and say "horse," but she never used the word in any context on her own. At bedtime one evening, Christopher walked out of her room shaking his head. He told me that Janie had just "read" him *Are You My Mother?* almost verbatim. Yet Janie would scream at the front door when she wanted to go out, even though she knew the word "outside."

When I would ask her, "Where's Sarah?" she looked at both of her siblings. She knew who Sarah and Luke were together, but did not know their names individually until well after she turned two.

One spring day a few months after her first EI evaluation, Janie and I were on a long walk when she counted to ten completely out of the blue from her stroller. I thought I had imagined it. Counting to ten tripled the total number of words she used at the time (aside from books and songs she memorized), and I had never heard her say a number before, although we had read plenty of counting books and listened to counting songs. She memorized every number from one to ten before she spoke any one of them aloud.

Janie observed, she memorized, she recited as she struggled to understand the world around her.

Happy Janie

Janie smiles as she wakes up. She windmills her arms while she runs. We have videos of her perched in her exersaucer laughing so hard at Luke's antics she could hardly catch her breath. Janie is naturally happy, a trait that attracted me to Christopher and one that happened to be a great antidote for her to inherit. Although Janie's disposition to an extent masked the disorder, her gregariousness and enthusiasm for life are two of her greatest assets in overcoming many of her symptoms of autism.

Wild Janie

With her exuberance also came a wild side. From birth, Janie had to go with the flow of her siblings' schedules. She never cried or objected when I woke her from a nap or interrupted play to buckle her into a car seat. Consequently, she exhibited less rigidity than typical of a child on the spectrum. Although when she had an opinion, she would not back down. I joked with Christopher that much like Texas, you don't mess with Janie. On the few things she felt strongly about, I did everything I could not to provoke her.

At dinner one night when Janie was not quite a year old, she was throwing her food all over the floor. When Sarah threw food as a toddler, I always admonished her, less so with Luke. By the time Janie went through the phase, I simply cleaned up the food without a word. Christopher was home for dinner that night and gently said, "No Janie, don't throw your food." She started crying, and Sarah and Luke jumped all over Christopher, "You can't say 'no' to Janie! That gets her upset!"

At the time, I saw their comments as eye opening to my own behavior, not bothering to correct her. Looking back, I also see that Janie's lack of communication skills prevented her from understanding why her behavior was curbed (less so than a typical one-year-old), which led to incredible frustration on her part, including brief, but highly acoustic tantrums.

I rarely took Janie to large grocery stores because she usually sat in the cart for less than five minutes before standing up and working on her escape. If I succumbed and let her out, she ran up and down the aisles ecstatic at her freedom, unresponsive to my requests for her to stay close to me. I ordered groceries online for a while, only taking the kids to a small, manageable grocery store that played calming music and had a spectacular candy aisle. Janie could be content eating Swedish fish and chocolate while I shopped.

But Sarah and Luke were not content. They had to wait until we checked out to have their candy. They also worried I would get in trouble for eating in the store and were usually on my case about it.

One day when Sarah was chastising me, I said, "Listen Sarah, I am five months pregnant with three kids at the grocery store, one who won't sit still in the cart unless I give her candy. So I'm giving her candy."

Sarah shot back, "Janie is a like a wild dog, and you need to train her." I burst out laughing and agreed. Janie was a bit wild, and we both needed some training.

Janie's Routines

Children with autism thrive on routine and predictability. Those tendencies started to emerge in Janie when she was one. She liked to go on her own adventures—and every adventure was the same. I let her take walks around the townhouses where we lived, following a step behind. She always took an identical route.

Janie headed out the front door, turned left onto the sidewalk, left again around the corner, and stopped at the first apartment building. There she pushed the numbers on the building's entry keypad before continuing on across the street. She hopped back up on the sidewalk, passed the playground and pool, and headed towards the gym. Then she would reach for my keys to open the door. We sometimes went inside to play with the giant exercise balls. She cried if we did not go in, and I would throw her up on my shoulders and swing her around until she was happy again. Then we retraced our steps back to the townhouse.

One day when Janie and I came home from grocery shopping, I locked the front door and ran upstairs to answer the phone. I chatted for a few minutes, unloading the groceries until I realized I could not hear Janie downstairs. I raced down, saw the door ajar, and sprinted out along her route—left out our door, left around the corner, nothing. I crossed the street with my heart in my mouth. Then I saw Janie by the playground up in the arms of a man clearly searching for a parent. I thanked him over and over, shaken to the core.

Janie's walking path was just one manifestation of her comfort in the familiarity of a routine. During the school year, we had the routine of her classes, naps, meals, and Sarah and Luke's schedules. The summer she turned two, we spent three weeks in Colorado with my parents. Towards the middle of the trip, Janie became feistier with more tantrums. At the time I could not understand why, but in hindsight I saw that the lack of predictability unsettled her. Janie's adherence to routine was one of the more subtle symptoms of autism that I did not pick up on initially.

Attached Janie

One of the main reasons I felt reluctant to set up the developmental evaluation was that Janie seemed so connected within our family. A hugger and a snuggler, she squeezed my head like a stuffed animal when I laid down with her at bedtime. Even in our extended family, Janie has always been affectionate.

She is number eight of 13 grandchildren on my side of the family. The older grandkids generally trail my father once they can swim, fish, or golf, but the toddlers usually ignored him—until Janie. With a house full of cousins running around, my father often settles on the floor to watch television, nap, or wrestle with the older ones. When Janie would see him there, she'd stop in her tracks, jump on his belly, and get wrapped up in a bear hug.

"Janie likes me!" he always yelled out. I think what she liked was his reservation around the younger kids, since he did not expect them to have any interest in him. She could initiate her interactions with my dad on her own terms. Some children on the spectrum are not comfortable with contact, while others crave it. I also learned later that squeezing soothed Janie.

Over several months following her EI evaluation, her attachment to family remained strong, but she gradually became reticent and detached around unfamiliar people. At her gym class each week when the teachers welcomed her in, Janie stopped whatever she was doing and stood motionless with her eyes shut. When they encouraged her to swing from the parallel bars or try a somersault, she refused. She cried if they held or even touched her. I pushed her to participate in the stations the teachers set up even if she was in hysterics, hoping she could move past her fear, which I realized later was a mistake.

The fall after she turned two, when I was still considering the developmental evaluation, Janie started up playcare one morning a week. She was familiar with my friend Cathy, who ran the playcare in her home and already knew three of the other five children who came on Tuesday mornings. Janie had become so attached to me over the summer, I warned Cathy that the transition might be tough for her. Cathy was not worried; she'd handled plenty of crying children.

Cathy encouraged me to stay with Janie the first day until she seemed comfortable. Janie wandered into Cathy's house, sticking close to me for about half an hour, checking out a few nearby toys, then venturing a bit further, coming to me for a hug every once in a while. At snack time, Janie sat with the other kids. Cathy asked each child if they would like water or apple juice, Pirates Booty or Goldfish. All the children answered but Janie, who smiled and looked away. After the kids went back to playing and Janie was engrossed in trains, I snuck out.

An hour and a half later, Cathy called. Janie had noticed me gone soon after I left and stood at the baby gate crying for me. Cathy could intermittently calm her down, but she was becoming more and more upset, I had better come back. When I pulled up, I could hear Janie crying from the driveway.

We tried again the following week. I stayed for the first half hour, then kissed Janie good-bye. She cried, so I stuck around. I left a little while later when she was happy playing with a toy. Cathy called after about 45 minutes; Janie was inconsolable. She had curled up sobbing next to a boy she knew. At that point, I understood something more was going on with Janie. If she was not ready to handle a new environment on her own, right or wrong, I would not continue to push her.

Janie and Other Kids

The boy Janie took comfort in at playcare was Billy. They had been in music class together for more than a year. They had also spent a morning together each week the previous school year while Billy's mom and I took turns volunteering in Luke and Billy's sister's Kindergarten classroom.

Billy adored Janie. He followed her around the house, showed her toys, tried to engage her in play, and asked her all sorts of questions. Janie completely ignored him. He didn't bother her; she seemed not to notice his entreaties at all. She regarded him more like an object than a person.

A few days before that first appointment with Dr. Shaw, we were swimming at the home of a friend whose son, Jack, was three weeks younger than Janie, but always three steps ahead of her in just about everything—crawling, walking, talking. If Janie had been my oldest, I may have found playing with Jack stressful. But by the time Janie came along, I had little concern with how she compared to her peers at such a young age, an attitude that contributed to my thinking of her issues as not that serious.

While Sarah and Luke went wild hopping from raft to raft, Janie stood on the steps of the pool with a tiny watering can filling and dumping cups over and over. Jack tried to engage Janie—saying her name repeatedly and then standing next to her with a matching watering can. Janie never even glanced at him. Eventually Jack took off in his floatie and played with Sarah and Luke instead.

Janie's World

That fall, Janie continued with her music class and also started ballet. She reveled in the outfits, the music, and staring at herself in the floor-to-ceiling mirror. She refused to stretch, hold anyone's hand besides mine, or crawl through the tunnel of mom legs. She sometimes followed the steps, but needed me to keep her on task. While the other girls sashayed along the hardwood floor, my daughter hung from the balance bar in her pink tutu with her spaghetti arms outstretched and knees bent to keep her ballet slippers from touching the ground—making monkey noises that echoed off the walls. She conducted her own ballet class parallel to the one going on around her.

Janie often played on her own for extended periods of time. I could help Sarah with homework, clean up the kitchen, fold laundry, answer emails—all with very little complaint from Janie, who looked at her books, listened to music, and sifted through the toy box in our sunroom. I attributed her independence to her being the third child.

Janie was an easy toddler, aside from her frustrations and stubbornness in certain situations. She engrossed herself in her own world. In a sense, she was disappearing into her mind and into her autism. I did not yet realize that we needed to pull her out of her inner world—and into the world around her.

3

EVALUATION

Post-Appointment

After Janie's visit with Dr. Shaw, the three kids and I met up with my friend Caren and her children at the beach. While the older kids played in the water and Janie sat on my lap snacking on crackers, I told Caren about the appointment and how it all seemed crazy to me. Did we really need to test Janie for autism? I was five months into a pregnancy with many complications. I felt spent, emotionally and physically.

The year before, we found out that Luke had some hearing loss. After a full workup, the ENT specialist explained to us the specific sounds he had difficulty hearing, and gave us advice on possible classroom accommodations and sports to avoid. She also recommended a CT scan, which would give us a 50/50 chance of determining the cause, genetic or environmental. Hearing loss is permanent and never improves; it either stays the same or worsens. I followed the doctor's advice to the letter, but kept harking back to the scan.

Should I put my five-year-old under anesthesia to possibly find out if his hearing would deteriorate further? I wavered for a few days, then cancelled the CT scan. Christopher agreed—we did not need the results of this test. We would address any future hearing loss when and if it occurs.

Caren had twins, a few months older than Janie, who were born 10 weeks early. From birth, they underwent tests and therapies non-stop. At a certain point, she went through with the tests and therapies she thought necessary and skipped the rest.

"The doctors thought I was wrong, but I know my children best. It was too much. I have no regrets," Caren said.

Plenty of kids talk late. Was this test really necessary?

I called my parents later that afternoon. Just as surprised as I had been at the suggestion Janie might have autism, they were somewhat at a loss for words and offered little advice. My mother was on the fence about the testing. She could not see the harm, but also knew I was wiped out by the pregnancy. My father said simply, "There's nothing wrong with Janie. She's perfect," and hopped off the phone.

I thought of the only person I knew with autism, my cousin Annie. I could not see any similarities between Janie and Annie. Only later did I recognize that Annie's symptoms were in fact very similar to Janie's, just more severe and pronounced. Janie being born a generation later than Annie drastically affected how differently their tendencies of autism would manifest. The services available to Annie and the understanding of autism at the time were light-years behind where they are today.

When Christopher came home that night, I told him about the appointment. Where I was perplexed, Christopher was unconcerned.

"I think Janie's fine. She's just taking her time talking. I'm not worried about her at all." So we shelved it for the time being.

Second Early Intervention Assessment

Although still unsure about the developmental evaluation

with Dr. Shaw, I felt strongly that Early Intervention would help Janie's speech progress. Ann Marie, from Janie's original EI assessment team, met with me first to get a better picture of Janie over the past year. I told her about Janie's strong personality, natural curiosity, love of music, playfulness with her brother and sister, and overall affection towards family members. I also explained Janie's timidness around new people. My primary concerns were her speech, temper, and ability to socialize with kids her age.

Ann Marie and I spoke at my kitchen table for about an hour while Janie roamed the house or played in the sunroom with a light-up alphabet game. She spent hours with this toy almost daily for about a month. Once she mastered all the letters and their sounds, she never touched it again.

"Does Janie always play so well by herself?" Ann Marie asked me.

"Yes, she's great at independent play," I said, considering her question a compliment until I noticed her watching Janie more closely. "Why? Is that unusual?"

"It's not typical for a child her age to play that long on their own without checking in with mom more often," said Ann Marie. Janie had swung by a few times for a hug and seemed perfectly content to me. And she was very content, in her own world.

"Does she answer to her name when you call her?" Ann Marie asked.

"Not usually, unless I have something she wants."

I silently began to question Ann Marie's questions. Everything she asked me was clearly significant, yet none were issues I had worried about.

"So how do you know if Janie is thirsty or hungry?"

"I guess I don't. I feed her at certain times and offer her water throughout the day."

"Does she ever point to food or her sippy cup to show you that she wants it?"

"No. Sometimes she just grabs food or a cup if she can reach it."

Ann Marie nodded, her expression unreadable. Her job was to determine Janie's needs for Early Intervention services, not to offer her thoughts on a diagnosis.

The following week, Ann Marie and her team conducted the Battelle Developmental Inventory. The same developmental therapist from the first evaluation drew Janie into our sunroom with toys to assess her skills. An hour and a half later, Janie's results were vastly different from the evaluation the previous year. A score of 77 or below in one or more areas qualify a child for EI services in our state. Seventy-seven was her top score among the categories.

Janie performed best on personal-social skills, which included her interaction with adults and peers, as well as her self-awareness and social development. I had described Janie as affectionate with family, but shy around new people, often looking away and hovering close to me. She clapped and smiled when praised and raised her arms to be picked up, although typically did not notice a person entering a room if playing.

Ann Marie noted in her report, "At times [Janie] will allow others to participate in her play. Today did not allow assessor to engage in play with her, moved away or picked another toy." Janie responded to directions inconsistently during the evaluation and did not identify herself in the mirror.

Janie scored a 73 for cognitive skills (how a child interacts with their environment, including attention, problem solving, and discrimination skills). When the therapist presented Janie with a toy, she usually made eye contact but would not engage, although she did uncover toys hidden under a blanket and played a shape sorting game. She did not pay attention to the book shown to her or reach for a toy behind a clear barrier. She pushed away nesting cups when offered, pulling out her own toys instead. Janie did seek me out during the assessment for comfort.

In motor development, Janie scored a 71, largely because she did not respond to tasks requested, such as jumping, picking up Cheerios, and drawing with a crayon. They also noticed that she did not point to anything, though she had been pointing at the 15-month assessment.

On adaptive skills (including feeding, dressing, hygiene, independence, and safety awareness), Janie scored a 70. They noted that she was a good eater, but did not use words or gestures to request food.

Janie scored the lowest on communication skills with a 55. She looked towards sounds (a bell ringing), but did not always respond to her name and did not look to me when asked, "Where's Mama?" Mainly quiet throughout the assessment, Janie sometimes babbled, sang, and repeated words spoken to her. She used words to label pictures in books, as well as letters and numbers, but not functionally (meaning communicatively). She did not use gestures or share joint attention, but instead fussed in front of a toy she wanted or simply reached for it herself.

Ann Marie summarized in the report, "Janie showed awareness of the new adults by turning away when approached. She settled with her mother on the floor of the playroom where the evaluation was administered. Janie was shown toys and objects in an attempt to engage her in play. She did establish eye contact and smiled slightly during a social/body play game, but otherwise maintained a neutral affect throughout the session. Janie showed initial interest in some of the toys (ring stack, dog pull toy, texture ball) and was noted to imitate some simple motor schemes ('wiggling' the dog's ears, 'poking' nubs on the texture ball, placing rings on the post). She also participated in an object permanence game (finding an animal figure when hidden under a cup). Janie turned away and engaged in her own activities much of the time. Her mother noted that she does tend to prefer to play alone rather than seeking others. Janie did involve her mother in play by attempting to give her a 'drink' from her toy teacup, and also pretending to sip it herself. She was noted to resist allowing the assessor to join her in this play, or to giving up her toys to the assessor. With regard to her language comprehension, Janie was not responsive to most verbal requests, however she did turn to her name today on two occasions and followed a direction to 'show it to Mama.' She responded to music with body movement and looked with increased interest to the assessor when she sang a familiar song. Expressively, Janie was often silent but when moving about on her own she was heard to babble and 'sing' tunefully. She also repeated some words spoken to her. Janie's lack of interest/ability to participate in many of the tasks clearly impacted her scores in some areas of this standardized tool. For example, she would not pick up Cheerios or a crayon, even though she is reported to feed herself and to color, therefore grasp patterns could not be scored; she was not able to imitate motor tasks such as jumping forward or throwing/kicking a ball, although she may be capable of demonstrating these skills spontaneously. Her motor skills did appear to be a strength."

Ann Marie would return the next week to discuss EI options for Janie.

Like Thomas

After meeting with the ladies from Early Intervention, I realized I needed to make up my mind on the autism evaluation. I had been leaning towards skipping it, but my feelings started to waver. I called a friend from college, Molly, whose son Thomas was three years older, but very similar to Janie.

As a toddler, Thomas seemed much more independent than Sarah and Luke. On vacation together one summer morning while making breakfast, I watched baby Thomas swatting a small water bottle across the kitchen floor and crawling after it. I commented to Molly how happy he was with a water bottle. She said he could go on like that for an hour, quite content on his own.

Thomas was often aloof—engrossed in his own world—and wary of unfamiliar adults, myself included. He screamed if I hugged him or tried to hold his hand, so I gave him his space. Although when Sarah and Luke chased and tackled him all over the house, he howled in delight.

Just after his second birthday, I watched him cuddled up on Molly's lap reading a book together. She opened tabs to find hidden letters, asking Thomas to name each one. He knew every letter and its sound. He could also count to ten in several languages. By four, he was reading Dr. Seuss books to Luke, who is a year older.

Yet Thomas had to be taught how to speak conversationally and to look people in the eye. He had an expressive language delay, although his receptive language was fine, meaning he could understand everything said to him, but had difficulty communicating to others. Thomas also had temper tantrums, particularly when away from home and his routine. The tantrums subsided as his communication skills progressed and the frustration of not being understood waned. He also started to warm up more easily around unfamiliar people.

Around age four, Thomas showed more interest in his peers, although he struggled relating to them. In karate class one day, Thomas tried to engage the child next to him by stepping on his foot. By five, he was polite, well-behaved, more comfortable with people outside his immediate family, easy to talk to, and played readily with other kids. His high intelligence set him apart a bit, but otherwise he was a typical five-year-old boy.

I knew that Thomas had Early Intervention services before he turned three and that he continued on with developmental and speech therapy into Kindergarten.

"I saw similarities between Janie and Thomas this summer," Molly said to me after I explained my quandary to her. We had all been out in Colorado together, where Janie had her share of temper tantrums. "Thomas used to get frustrated just like Janie before he could talk."

I told her about Janie's appointment with Dr. Shaw and the Early Intervention evaluation.

"Janie's eval sounds exactly like Thomas'," she said. "He was constantly singing and memorized everything. He didn't respond to his name. He played by himself all the time and became angry so easily."

Before Thomas turned two, Molly expressed concern to her pediatrician, who assured her that a speech delay was not out of the ordinary. They moved a few months later, and the new pediatrician agreed with Molly that the speech delay was significant enough to warrant Early Intervention. By the time Thomas was evaluated and assigned therapists, he had only three months left before aging out of the program. They then found speech and developmental therapists for Thomas. He was tested for autism and other developmental disorders, but not given a diagnosis.

"Janie has been late to do everything—rolling, sitting, walking. If it's probably just a speech delay, do you think this test is really necessary?" I asked her.

"If I were you, I would definitely do the evaluation."

Janie was so much like Thomas, who did not have autism—I was surprised Molly thought we should.

"You want Janie to get the therapy she needs to address any delays," she told me. "And there's a chance she might be diagnosed with PDD-NOS."

This conversation was not going the way I expected. "PDD-what?"

"PDD-NOS. Pervasive Developmental Disorder Not Otherwise Specified. The doctor didn't diagnose Thomas with PDD-NOS, but we practically begged him to."

"Why would you want him to have a diagnosis?"

"A diagnosis opens a lot of doors. With or without it, Thomas needed developmental and speech therapy. We spent hours on the phone with our insurance company and paid for much of his therapy out of pocket. But it made all the difference in the world for Thomas."

I went silent, mulling over her advice.

"You caught whatever is going on early. I wish we had realized sooner that Thomas needed therapy." The last thing she said was the clincher for me. "A lot hardwires between two and three."

I set up the evaluation with Dr. Shaw as soon as we hung up.

Therapy Begins

Luke and Sarah started up first and third grade in September. Janie cried each morning when they rode away on the bus and was ecstatic when they hopped off the bus in the afternoons. By the second week, the tears stopped when she realized they would always return to her.

That fall Janie's days were filled with playdates, walks outside, music and ballet classes, and soon enough, therapy. Soccer season began for Sarah and Luke, and much to Janie's delight, Sarah also started playing the violin.

Ann Marie came by the week following Janie's EI evaluation to go over their recommendations. I expected her to assign Janie a speech therapist. Instead Ann Marie suggested a developmental therapist.

"I have a therapist in mind who I think would be a great match for Janie and for you," Ann Marie said. "Her name is Megan. She has a private practice and contracts with EI. She could work with Janie up to six hours a week."

"Six hours? I was thinking Janie would have one or two hours a week of therapy."

"Well, let's start with two and see what you and Megan think she needs."

I agreed, my mind racing to figure out where we would find six hours a week for Early Intervention between Janie's activities and afternoon naps, plus balancing Sarah and Luke's schedules. I pushed aside other disquieting thoughts.

Megan called a few days later. On the phone she was cheerful and accommodating to Janie's schedule. From her tone and manner, I pictured a twenty-something girl, fresh off her schooling and full of energy. On the sunny Monday morning when Megan showed up at our door, I was surprised to see she was about my age. She had thick, dark red hair cut just below her chin, with bangs blanketing her forehead. Megan's smile was ear-to-ear, and she carried more bags than seemed possible, all spilling over with toys. I think often of that late September day meeting Megan for the first time, having no idea of the impact she would have on Janie's life.

Megan knew not to come on strong with Janie. She said "Hi" and waved, then hung back, talking to me until Janie eventually approached her. Megan told me about her practice and background. Not exactly fresh out of grad school, Megan had almost 25 years of experience. She had a general family practice and specialized in helping children on the autism spectrum and kids dealing with anxiety and other social and communication issues.

Megan was trained in the Early Start Denver Model (ESDM), a therapy for children with autism from 12 to 48 months of age. ESDM focuses on developing a child's social-emotional, cognitive, and language skills and takes an integrative approach to reaching specific, measurable goals through play.[1] Therapies are somewhat geographic; Megan was the only ESDM therapist in our state at the time.

In an hour and a half, Megan and Janie played dolls, peek-a-boo, and Play-Doh, stacked and crashed blocks, read books, and dropped toy cars down slides. Janie was reserved, but interacted with Megan, imitating her play and intermittently speaking a few single words. That first day, Megan suggested I talk to Janie in one- to two-word phrases for easier comprehension, while facing her so that she could see my expressions.

The next morning, Megan was back for another session. She sang "Old MacDonald," coaxing Janie into singing along and holding her interest with accompanying finger plays. They also played with Little People and Play-Doh again. Megan blew bubbles, and Janie followed her directions to clap or stomp them.

When Janie ran from Megan, ignored her, or became upset, my maternal instinct kicked in to intervene or entreat her to come back, but Megan let me know that she was used to everything—from disinterest to tantrums. During therapy sessions, she would be the one to get Janie's attention, keep her interest, and deal with inappropriate behavior. Janie could come to me for hugs and reassurance. So I learned to simply observe unless Megan asked for my participation.

During the first weeks of therapy, Janie often sat on my lap or next to me while she played with Megan. Eventually I moved to a chair a few feet away, and then a bit farther when Janie felt comfortable enough with Megan to not need the security of me nearby.

Therapy was not what I anticipated. It looked simply like play to me. Megan's animated gestures and speech brought an atmosphere of excitement and fun to the sessions, and Janie seemed to enjoy their interactions. Who wouldn't want a playmate like Megan? The first few sessions, I thought Megan was solely focused on building a rapport with Janie, but soon realized that every activity Megan did with her had a therapeutic purpose.

Megan often playfully chased Janie to engage her back in play, as she usually participated in an activity for only a few minutes before wandering away. In those early weeks, Megan established familiar routines and began to teach essential skills, many of which I had not realized Janie lacked.

• • •

Janie's Neurobehavioral Evaluation

Dr. Shaw met with Janie twice in September for about two hours each time. We came directly after ballet class, Janie in her pink leotard and tutu. She and Dr. Shaw zoomed balloons around the room, stacked blocks, played with *Sesame Street* characters, fitted shape sorters, played peek-a-boo, nested cups, matched objects and pictures, and had a birthday party with little cups, plates, and a pretend cake.

Through this play, Dr. Shaw conducted the Autism Diagnostic Observation Schedule to assess Janie's social and communication skills, and the Mullen Scales of Early Learning to measure her cognitive abilities.

Surprisingly, Janie was fairly happy to play with Dr. Shaw, who clearly had the touch engaging with children like her. Aside from one test towards the end of the first session when she lost her patience matching pictures, Janie enjoyed all the toys and activities. Dr. Shaw asked me if I thought she had seen all of Janie's skills once the evaluation was complete, and I did for the most part. Janie was responsive and behaved as she usually did throughout the testing.

During these evaluations, I picked up on more clues that a diagnosis was a real possibility. When I described Janie's involved play with Sarah and Luke, Dr. Shaw countered that her older siblings made it easy for Janie—they catered to her needs and preferences, whereas interacting with a peer her own age took much more understanding on her part. When Janie held Bert and Ernie figures in each of her hands, Dr. Shaw asked me if she often carried two objects. Yes, she liked comparing similar toys and books. Dr. Shaw nodded as she jotted down notes.

Once we finished up the assessment, we scheduled a meeting a month out to go over the results. In the meantime, I asked Megan if she thought Janie would be diagnosed with a disorder.

Megan took her time with her answer. She began by telling me that while qualified to make a diagnosis, she worked with Janie as her Early Intervention therapist, so was not in a position to do so. "Regardless of whether or not Janie gets a diagnosis, it won't change who she is."

I understood Megan's professionalism. I also understood that she was preparing me, and that surprised me.

She explained that Dr. Shaw tested Janie for five Pervasive Developmental Disorders. "The only diagnosis that might apply to Janie is PDD-NOS. I don't know if she will be diagnosed. A lot depends on the doctor."

I told her how Molly had wanted a diagnosis for her son.

"Having a diagnosis will give Janie the option of more services. You really want as much therapy as you can get for her."

Ann Marie came by to check in a few days before my appointment with Dr. Shaw. She asked me if I was sure I wanted the results of the evaluation the week before I was due. "If Janie does end up getting a diagnosis, it may be a lot to handle all at once with a new baby."

I knew my life would be turned upside down once the baby arrived, and I needed to get a grip on this before the chaos. Ann Marie simply asking me that question further added to my expectation of a diagnosis. (EI therapists and supervisors can recommend an evaluation for a child, but cannot give or speculate on a diagnosis.)

"In the event that Janie does have a diagnosis, Dr. Shaw will most likely recommend ABA therapy. You should think about whether you'd like to stick with Megan or do ABA. You'd get more hours of therapy if you go with ABA, but with Megan you could continue with ESDM therapy." Ann Marie went on to explain ABA in more detail and tried to hold back from pushing me either way, but I could see she thought I should choose quality over quantity. "You just don't find many therapists like Megan."

I didn't need convincing.

4

DIAGNOSIS AND AUTISM 101

A Diagnosis for Janie

"Don't you want your husband to be here?" Dr. Shaw asked me as we sat down at a table in the room full of toys where she had tested Janie.

Christopher had offered to take off work, but by now I knew what was coming. I had slowly absorbed the shock of an impending diagnosis over the past few weeks. Dr. Shaw first suggesting the evaluation got me thinking, but Ann Marie's questions and suggestions about Janie's behavior indicated to me that she also suspected more than just developmental delays.

In the four weeks of therapy with Megan prior to the diagnosis, I started to see Janie in ways I never had before. I had my first glimpses into her world and realized how differently her mind worked. I was genuinely surprised at Megan's response when I asked her opinion about a diagnosis, but I knew she understood Janie better than I did. My feelings had been shifting on the likelihood of a diagnosis for Janie, and after our conversation the shift was complete.

My older brother inadvertently gave me some simple advice that I often fall back on when coming to terms with life not turning out how I imagined. A few months before Janie was diagnosed, he separated from his wife. When I asked how he was doing, he talked about the pain the separation caused his kids and the loneliness of coming home to an empty apartment, but overall he was doing well and felt it was the right decision. He also mentioned that he did not like people saying how sorry they were for him. He never seemed to feel sorry for himself. "It is what it is," he said.

After realizing Janie would have a diagnosis, I thought about my pregnancy with her. *Was I too old? Was I too stressed? Did we live too close to that cell tower?* I worried about Janie. *Would she make friends? Would she have a full life?* With everything that fell on our lap that year, I knew I could not get mired in those thoughts. I told myself constantly: *It is what it is*.

Dr. Shaw began the conversation by explaining her concerns that prompted the evaluation for Janie: language delays, including her small vocabulary (unless singing or reciting books), and not calling people by name or attempting to communicate; social delays, specifically her limited eye contact and interest in kids her age; and behavioral concerns, such as her issues with transitions. In her report, Dr. Shaw wrote, "Janie's performance was notable for difficulty with reciprocal and social interactions, communication, and repetitive behaviors," which pretty much sums up a child on the autism spectrum.

During the assessment, Janie did have occasional eye contact with Dr. Shaw and sometimes responded to her name, but showed very little joint attention (at least that coordinated eye contact, pointing, and language). Dr. Shaw noted in her report, "Quality of social overtures was slightly unusual and usually restricted to personal demands or strong interests. Many times Janie attempted to get things she wanted by herself."

Janie only said five words and one two-word phrase ("Bye bubbles") during the entire evaluation. She jargoned (using unintelligible language) and echoed Dr. Shaw a few times.

Her play was often repetitive and not as functional as typical of her age. Dr. Shaw also noticed "mild signs of anxiety and negativism" and that Janie sometimes walked on her tippy-toes, strangely enough a common symptom for children on the spectrum.

On the positive side, she noted that, "Janie's cognition/problem-solving skills were largely appropriate for chronological age, which is a wonderful strength."

While Janie had significant social and communication impairments, as well as repetitive and restricted behaviors, they were more mild than severe. Dr. Shaw diagnosed her with PDD-NOS.

The only part of the discussion that did shock me—which in hindsight, baffles me how I missed it—was that PDD-NOS is on the autism spectrum. I had thought that autism, Asperger's Disorder, and PDD-NOS were mainly unrelated, aside from being developmental disorders.

I explained my confusion to Dr. Shaw, and she went over each again. In my mind, Janie still did not have autism; she was just on the spectrum. I was not 100 percent there, but getting closer.

"So what do I need to do?" Now that the diagnosis was official, I needed a plan.

Dr. Shaw recommended 20 hours a week of intensive one-on-one behavioral therapy, both ABA and Floortime, focusing on "social reciprocity, communication, imitation, joint attention, and play skills," in addition to speech and possibly occupational therapy.

My mind was reeling. How would we fit in that much therapy? I could hardly keep all the kids' fingernails clipped. When would she nap?

"Is speech therapy included in that 20 hours?" I finally got out.

"No, that would be an additional hour each week."

I know how fortunate I am to live in a state that would allow us 20 hours a week of therapy virtually free of charge—

and how critical it is for a child with autism to receive intensive therapy at such a young age, but logistically, I had a baby due the following week, plus two other children to figure in. This much therapy did not seem physically possible.

"I don't know that we can feasibly do 20 hours a week. How many hours would you be happy with?" I worded it terribly, but I wanted to do what was best for Janie and be realistic.

Dr. Shaw was less familiar with ESDM therapy, but after I explained Janie's relationship with and my confidence in Megan, she agreed that 10 hours a week of therapy with Megan in lieu of ABA and Floortime, as well as an hour of speech therapy each week, would be fine.

Then I asked her the question I knew she could not answer: "What will Janie be like when she's older?"

Dr. Shaw let out her breath and said, "I wish I had a crystal ball that I could look into and tell you. It's impossible to say. The two biggest factors in treating autism are catching it early and intensive therapy. Janie has both going for her."

I called Christopher after the appointment. I had told him earlier that Janie would most likely get a diagnosis. He was not upset now that it was a reality, but he disagreed. He thought Janie had speech and other delays, and that therapy with Megan was necessary, but Janie was not on the autism spectrum. He felt as I had initially. Although he watched a few therapy sessions and read all the session notes, not seeing Janie regularly with Megan and kids her age, he did not fully understand her deficits. Her vivacity and spirit also belied her diagnosis—she did not fit his perception of autism. In time, he did change his mind.

As for me, I did not mourn the diagnosis long. Janie's world was a new world to me. I would immerse myself in it to help her as best I could.

Finn's Arrival

Exactly one week after receiving Janie's diagnosis, her brother Finn was born. Christopher and I left for the hospital before sunrise. My in-laws stayed with the kids for the five days I was away. The C-section went smoothly, and we had a healthy little baby boy.

I had read Janie the big sister/new baby books and talked to her about the baby in my tummy, but had little indication how much registered with her. Christopher brought Sarah and Luke to visit me in the hospital, but not Janie. I did not want to confuse and upset her since I wouldn't be coming home with them. She enjoyed her time with her grandparents without any issues until the third and fourth days, when she repeatedly asked for me.

Sarah and Luke did not know if they had a new brother or sister until they came to the hospital. Christopher let "she" slip a few times on the drive in to throw them off, although Luke was fairly confident the baby would be a boy to fit the girl-boy pattern we had going. I held Finn up for them when they came into the room. They looked at the baby perplexed until I let out, "It's a boy!" Luke hollered, "Yes!"

While Sarah and Luke could not wait to get their little brother home, I worried how Janie would react to Finn—she had become a bit possessive of me. On a few occasions swimming together over the summer, if Sarah and Luke held onto me in the pool, Janie peeled them off. In her stroller, if she turned and saw one of them pushing her, she screamed until I took over. She also voiced her objections when Luke or Sarah hugged me.

Janie's reaction to Finn was completely unexpected in that she had no reaction. She seemed not to notice him at all. When I nursed Finn, she climbed over him as if he were an inanimate object. She plucked pacifiers out of his mouth for herself like he was a doll. While plenty of typical kids might ignore a new sibling, Janie took months to acknowledge her brother. Finn was a complete nonentity to her, which I found more upsetting than the expected jealousy. Her reaction confirmed to me again that Janie was not like other children.

Accepting Autism

For a few months, I thought of PDD-NOS as separate from autism, even though I understood it to be on the spectrum. When I talked about her diagnosis with close friends and relatives they would sometimes ask, "But she doesn't have autism?" Most adults think of *Rain Man* when they hear the word autism. And on the surface, Janie did not seem anything like *Rain Man.*

I would say unwittingly, "No, she's on the autism spectrum, but she has PDD-NOS. Not autism." Then I would explain PDD-NOS as best I could. Finally, I started to question my assumption. I asked Megan if she thought Janie had autism.

Megan was thoughtful in her answer. "In this part of the country, people use the term PDD-NOS. In other parts of the country, people call it mild autism. PDD-NOS and mild autism are the same thing. It's just terminology."

Christopher shrugged his shoulders when I talked to him about it that evening. "I think everything we're doing for Janie is exactly what she needs, and I have complete confidence in Megan. Janie has delays, but she doesn't have autism."

I did not argue with Christopher, but I disagreed. He needed time. I accepted what Megan told me, although I needed some time too. Aside from Christopher, I kept it to myself for a while. I needed to wrap my head around this word now applied to my daughter and come to terms myself with the fact that she had autism. In a few weeks, I would move on. How could I feel sorry for myself or Janie when her symptoms were not severe? She was flagged early and making great progress with an amazing therapist. It is what it is.

Once I felt settled myself with the autism moniker, I talked to my parents about it over the phone. Neither of them got it. When they thought of people with autism, like Temple Grandin or my cousin Annie, they could not make the connection to Janie. Plus, she had so much spirit and affection, her detachment from the world around her could be difficult to perceive. My mother struggled to understand, but accepted it. My father disagreed and repeated what he said earlier, "Janie's perfect."

Several weeks later my parents came for a visit. My father took Janie to her ballet class. When they arrived home, Janie burst through the front door in her tutu, and my dad shuffled in behind her. I asked him how it went as we watched Janie pull out toys in the sunroom. He looked me in the eyes and said, "Watching her with the other little girls, I saw it. I saw the difference. I understand now."

My mother-in-law visits us a couple of times a month, a flurry of energy and positivity. She has a deep connection with my kids and somehow manages to spend time with each one while also washing, folding, and putting away all our laundry and tidying up anything out of place. I have never seen her raise her voice or show the slightest irritation. She is one of the most selfless people I know.

She sometimes watched Megan's sessions and always remarked at how well Janie was doing. She had early on wanted to clarify that Janie did not have autism. I sat her down one day to explain how I had misunderstood her diagnosis. I could see her eyes welling with tears as I spoke, and I found myself echoing Megan.

"It doesn't change who she is. Janie is still the same person." I talked about the strides she had made already, but did not have answers for how Janie would look in the future. She held back her emotions, but I could see she was crushed. She did not want Janie to struggle or suffer.

She read up on autism, asked often about Janie's progress and therapy, and was not crushed for long. My mother-in-law is everyone's cheerleader, and Janie was no exception.

I have been careful choosing what to tell Sarah and Luke about Janie's disorder. I describe her challenges and how we can help her, but I have yet to use the word autism. It took me months to understand how she fit on the spectrum. Emotionally and intellectually, they need more time.

Christopher and I debated often whether or not Janie had autism. He would focus on a single symptom, like talking late or memorizing books, and asked where the line was between delays and autism. And the line can be murky—that is why so much of a diagnosis depends on the doctor and why the diagnoses keep changing. Plenty of typical kids meticulously arrange their toys or flap their arms when excited. How extreme these characteristics are and whether age appropriate need to be taken into consideration.

The symbol for autism is interlocking puzzle pieces. Taken in isolation, symptoms of autism can be found in any child. Like the puzzle, put together those symptoms can indicate autism. All of Janie's delays collectively set her on the spectrum. Her repetitive behaviors, sensory sensitivities, and more significantly, social and communication deficits taken as a whole pointed to autism.

History of Diagnosing Autism

Derived from the Greek word "autos" which means "self," autism was first defined in the beginning of the 20th century by Swiss psychiatrist, Eugen Bleuler, as "withdrawal into one's inner world."[1] Bleuler considered autism a form of schizophrenia.

In 1943, an American child psychiatrist, Dr. Leo Kanner, was the first to flesh out autism as a disorder in a paper describing his studies of 11 children of high intelligence whose "activities and utterances are governed rigidly and consistently by the powerful desire for aloneness and sameness."[2] The following year, Austrian psychologist Hans Asperger, published a paper relating the characteristics of what later became known as Asperger's Disorder.[3]

Several decades passed before autism was understood as it is today and treated with effective therapies. The first Diagnostic and Statistical Manual of Mental Disorders (DSM-I) was published by the American Psychiatric Association in 1952 to describe and classify mental disorders. DSM-I categorized autism as "schizophrenic reaction, childhood type."[4]

During the 1960s, many believed in the "refrigerator mother" theory that colder, more withdrawn mothers caused autism. In the 1970s, scientists recognized autism's biological roots, and that it derives from the brain rather than parenting styles.[5]

DSM-III finally separated autism from schizophrenia in 1980 and included the newly termed, "Pervasive Developmental Disorder."[6] Seven years later, DSM-III-R offered a fuller checklist of symptoms to diagnose "Autistic Disorder," as well as the PDD-NOS diagnosis.[7] Treatment shifted to behavioral therapy.

DSM-IV and DSM-IV-TR, published in 1994 and 2000 respectively, further defined Autistic Disorder, classified under the encompassing category of Pervasive Developmental Disorders, which also included Asperger's Disorder, PDD-NOS, Rett Syndrome, and Childhood Disintegrative Disorder.[8][9]

In 2013, DSM-5 changed the entire classification of autism.[10]

Autism Spectrum Disorders

Pervasive Developmental Disorders (PDDs) refer to a group of disorders that share impairments in development related to social interaction and communication skills, as well as repetitive and rigid patterns of behavior.[11] Socially, individuals with PDDs are characterized by deficits in sharing emotions, understanding others' perspectives and feelings, showing empathy, or in communicating.[12] Children with PDD struggle with both verbal and nonverbal communication, including pointing, gestures, and eye contact.[13] A child's interests are often restricted and highly focused.[14] According to the Autism Consortium, "PDDs are called 'spectrum' disorders because each child has symptoms that differ in intensity, ranging from mild to quite severe."[15]

Of the five PDDs, three were considered Autism Spectrum Disorders (ASDs).[16] The first, Autistic Disorder, often referred to as "classic" autism,[17] is what might come to mind when a layperson thinks of autism. A child with Autistic Disorder has significant deficits in behavioral, social, and communication skills.[18] A child with Pervasive Developmental Disorder Not Otherwise Specified (PDD-NOS) has challenges in some but not all of these areas and in a milder form than a child with Autistic Disorder.[19]

As defined by DSM-IV-TR, people with Asperger's Disorder do not have delays in speech development and have strong basic language skills, but struggle in social situations and in reciprocal conversation. They also tend to have fixated interests and behavioral issues.[20]

The other two PDDs are less common. Rett Syndrome, now known to be an identifiable genetic disorder, causes a child to lose motor skills, especially hand use.[21] Childhood Disintegrative Disorder becomes apparent around age three or four when a child's communication, social, play, and motor skills suddenly begin to disappear.[22]

DSM-5 Shakes Up the Spectrum

In 2013 (after Janie was diagnosed), DSM-5 significantly changed the criteria for autism and eliminated the monikers, Asperger's Disorder and PDD-NOS, altogether.[23] These two disorders, in addition to Autistic Disorder and Childhood Disintegrative Disorder, are now all considered Autism Spectrum Disorder or ASD.[24] The other PDD, Rett Syndrome, is no longer classified as an ASD.[25]

DSM-5 describes Autism Spectrum Disorder as "persistent deficits in social communication and social interaction" and "restricted, repetitive patterns of behavior."[26] Symptoms of ASD impact a child's personal relationships, "ranging, for example, from difficulties adjusting behavior to suit various social contexts; to difficulties in sharing imaginative play or in making friends; to absence of interest in peers."[27] Also affected are nonverbal communication skills, such as eye contact. Symptoms may additionally include: "Stereotyped or repetitive motor movements, use of objects, or speech…Insistence on sameness…Highly restricted, fixated interests… Hyper- or hyporeactivity to sensory input or unusual interests in sensory aspects of the environment."[28]

To distinguish where a child's symptoms fall along the spectrum, a severity level always follows the Autism Spectrum Disorder diagnosis: Level 1 ("requiring support"), Level 2 ("requiring substantial support"), or Level 3 ("requiring very substantial support").[29] The diagnosis may also include a specifier: ASD with or without accompanying intellectual impairment; ASD with or without accompanying language impairment; ASD associated with a known medical or genetic condition or environmental factor; ASD associated with another neurodevelopmental, mental, or behavioral disorder; or ASD with catatonia.[30]

DSM-5 also introduced a new diagnosis separate from ASD, called Social (Pragmatic) Communication Disorder (SCD), characterized by "persistent difficulties in the social use of verbal and nonverbal communication."[31] A person with SCD might struggle with greeting people, participating in a conversation appropriately, understanding the nuances of speaking in different contexts, interpreting body language, and overall engaging in social relationships.[32] A child with SCD has less severe social impairments than a child with ASD and no repetitive behaviors or sensory issues.[33]

DSM-5 clearly states that diagnoses of Autistic Disorder, Asperger's Disorder, and PDD-NOS should be changed to ASD or SCD, although the doctors and therapists I have spoken with firmly expressed that those diagnosed prior to DSM-5 could keep their original diagnoses, particularly if they identify with them.

Treatments for Autism

Doctors typically recommend up to 30 hours of services each week for children diagnosed with autism. If diagnosed under the age of three, a child qualifies for Early Intervention (EI).[34] Although the name may vary, EI is offered in every state. Insurance companies and state governments usually pick up the bulk of the cost. For the first six months of Janie's EI services, we paid $150 total. Since then our state laws have changed so that there is no cost at all.

EI offers developmental therapy, speech therapy, occupational therapy, physical therapy, group therapy, and sometimes music therapy. They can also provide a social worker, nutritionist, nurse, or psychotherapist. Specialists come to a child's home or daycare to provide services.[35]

Megan contracted through Early Intervention and practiced ESDM therapy with Janie. Applied Behavior Analysis (ABA) and Floortime are also common therapies for autism.[36] ABA is very structured, repeatedly working on specific skills by breaking them down into small steps with a reward system to reinforce mastery.[37] Floortime centers on play and following the child's lead to teach social and communication skills.[38]

Other specialty services for children with autism include Pivotal Response Treatment (PRT), Verbal Behavior (VB) therapy, Relationship Development Intervention (RDI), Training and Education of Autistic and Related Communication Handicapped Children (TEACCH), and Social Communication/Emotional Regulation/Transactional Support (SCERTS), among many others.

Developmental therapy is not a one size fits all solution. While we never tried other autism-specific therapies, I have no doubt that ESDM was the best therapy for Janie. A more withdrawn child, less responsive to social rewards, might make the most progress with ABA, for example. Interestingly enough, the therapy a family chooses for their child often depends upon where they live and the therapies available in that area.

Once a child turns three, they age out of Early Intervention. Responsibility for therapeutic service delivery then moves to the town's department of education.[39] Therapy usually takes place at a local school, although home services are sometimes offered as well.[40]

The Early Start Denver Model of Therapy

The Early Start Denver Model (ESDM) is a behavioral therapy for younger children (12 to 48 months old) diagnosed on the autism spectrum. Developed by psychologists Sally Rogers and Geraldine Dawson, ESDM lays out a set of skills for a child to acquire and a curriculum to teach these skills in a natural setting, typically the child's home.[41] The family is integrally involved, so that therapy continues beyond the sessions. ESDM therapy focuses heavily on a child's relationships and increasing skills in social-emotional, cognitive, and language areas using regular assessments of progress to tailor the program to the individual child.[42]

ESDM therapy can be loosely described as a model that blends components of ABA, the original Denver Model, and Pivotal Response Treatment into an integrated approach to intervention. While ABA emphasizes working on each goal discretely, ESDM often tackles many facets at once, such as playing a game that involves turn-taking, making eye contact, and following two-step directions. Similar to Floortime,

ESDM teaches social and communication skills through play routines, but is much more data-based (with the therapist recording progress and checking goals every 15 minutes), and the curriculum for therapy is individualized to the child.

In the United States, ESDM has a presence in Arizona, California, Colorado, Connecticut, Florida, Georgia, Illinois, Indiana, Kansas, Maine, Massachusetts, Michigan, Minnesota, Missouri, Nevada, New Hampshire, New Jersey, New York, North Carolina, Pennsylvania, Tennessee, Texas, Utah, Vermont, Virginia, Washington, and Wisconsin. Internationally, ESDM therapists are available in Australia, Austria, Azerbaijan, Belgium, Brazil, Canada, the Cayman Islands, China, Denmark, France, Germany, Greece, Ireland, Israel, Italy, Japan, Kuwait, Mexico, Nepal, New Zealand, Poland, Portugal, Saudi Arabia, South Africa, South Korea, Spain, Sweden, Switzerland, Taiwan, Thailand, United Arab Emirates, and Vietnam. A full list of ESDM therapists can be found on the University of California at Davis MIND Institute's web site at www.esdm.co.

Accessibility varies widely. Drs. Rogers and Dawson published a book called *An Early Start for your Child with Autism,* that details ESDM activities parents can do with their children.[43] *Implementing the Group-Based Early Start Denver Model for Preschoolers with Autism,* by Giacomo Vivanti and Ed Duncan, is an excellent resource for teachers and professionals providing services to young children on the autism spectrum.[44]

PART II

INTENSIVE THERAPY (JANIE FROM 2 – 2½ YEARS OLD)

5

ESDM THERAPY

Therapy Ramps Up

As September passed into October and November, Sarah and Luke often asked about Megan, whom they had yet to meet since she came while they were at school. Sarah and Luke were too young to understand the concept of autism, so I explained that she was helping Janie learn to talk and have less tantrums. Megan slowly added in more time with Janie each week, and by December, we were up to two hours of therapy four mornings a week.

During the sessions, I usually sat on the couch in our living room watching Megan and Janie together while Finn nursed or slept on my lap. Our house has an open floor plan —the front door leads into the living room with a sunroom straight ahead and kitchen off to the left. It is not a large house, but its sunny openness does make it feel bigger.

I started to catch on after several therapy sessions. Driving past Megan one day in town, I thought she looked sad behind the wheel. Passing another car, I realized she had the same affect as the next driver—I had simply never seen Megan in downtime, not overly animated while teaching a two-year-old with autism how to socialize. Her exaggerated gestures demonstrated to Janie expressions that match words and emotions, as well as their meanings, while also encouraging her to gesture herself.

Slowly beginning to see how little I understood about Janie, my questions for Megan piled up during the sessions. I did not want to interrupt Janie's therapy, but Megan seemed to get my daughter in ways that I did not. Her depth of experience, natural instincts, and intelligence brought me answers that were spot on, well thought out, and tremendously helpful.

I tried to hold my questions in until Janie's short breaks when Megan recorded data, then let them burst out. I wanted clarity and advice. Megan did not explain the purpose of every activity they did, but peppered the sessions with suggestions to help Janie progress. Soon I was taking notes.

ESDM and Janie's PDD-NOS

ESDM does not take a turnkey approach to therapy. Megan was not treating PDD-NOS in general, she treated *Janie's* PDD-NOS. To begin with, she checked in regularly with me about Janie's sleeping, eating, her participation in community programs, and anything else going on in her life, so that she had a full picture to consider. If Janie's sleep had been off, for instance, Megan would not push too hard in therapy, giving her ample breaks.

Janie's therapy was customized to her particular symptoms. Megan utilized Janie's strengths to ameliorate her weaknesses. For example, Janie is a master imitator, verbally and physically. Megan and our family constantly modeled words and phrases that belong to different situations, such as "Good catch!" after throwing a ball. Janie memorized those phrases until they became natural for her.

Megan followed Janie's lead in play. She brought plenty of toys, but did not have an agenda of toys to play with—only an agenda of goals. If the goal was teaching Janie to take turns, and

Janie veered toward Play-Doh instead of the "Sorry!" game she had pulled out, Megan would say, "Oh, you want to do Play-Doh," and they would take turns with the roller. Megan did not always do what Janie wanted her to; in fact, as they worked on easing Janie's rigidity, she sometimes did not follow Janie's lead if she became too controlling over how a game should be played.

ESDM therapists continually approach symptoms in new ways until they are minimized or eliminated. While ESDM suggests many activities to elicit certain skills from a child, the therapy is also designed to be off the cuff in finding novel solutions to fit a child's interests or a situation. For example, Janie's tendency to hold a toy in each hand sometimes restricted her from fully participating in an activity. During one session, she had a toy giraffe in one hand and a bear in the other, refusing to part with either. Megan sat the animals on a tiny toy couch to "watch" Janie work at the easel, which delighted her.

Goals

During the first few sessions, Megan conducted an ESDM assessment of Janie, which again to me looked purely like play. Based on the results, she developed a specific set of goals from the ESDM curriculum tailored to Janie and recorded data throughout their sessions to track those goals. She would assess Janie again when she achieved most of those milestones or up to 12 weeks later, then develop new goals in accordance with her progress. Following are Janie's first set of objectives:

Receptive Communication:

RC:1:6 During a playful interaction, when an adult states, "Janie, look" while holding an interesting object, Janie will turn her head and look at the object 3 times within an hour session, with at least 2 different adults, across 3 out of 4 consecutive sessions.

RC:1:8 When a play partner points proximally to indicate an object or location, Janie will follow gesture and turn head toward indicated direction of object or location for 4 of 5 opportunities with 2 play partners across 3 consecutive sessions.

RC:1:10 During a social game, Janie will attend and respond to adult gestures or words by looking, reaching, gesturing, or smiling for 1 or more rounds with 2 or more adults for 3 consecutive days (games: peekaboo, Where is Thumbkin, high five routines).

Expressive Communication:

EC:1:7 Janie will make eye contact to obtain a desired object when an adult blocks or withholds access to the object 5 times in 45 minutes, with 2 adults, across 3 consecutive sessions.

EC:1:8 When offered a choice of objects, Janie will use her index finger to point to indicate preferred object at least 3 times during 15 minutes of play with 2 or more play partners for 3 consecutive days.

Social Skills:

SS:1:4 +7 During familiar sensory social routines, Janie will maintain engagement with a play partner for at least 2 minutes and will participate at least 2 or more times with any active behavior such as making eye contact, reaching, imitating, vocalizing within the routine with at least 2 different people within at least 5 sensory social routines or songs across 3 out of 4 consecutive sessions.

SS:1:6 When engaged in parallel play with adult and adult models play action, Janie will participate within 5 seconds by imitating at least 2 play actions to continue play for 3 parallel play activities across 3 consecutive sessions, 2 settings, and 2 play partners.

Imitation:

I:1:1 When an adult gains Janie's attention and models a one-step action on object, Janie will imitate 8 one-step actions on objects within 5 seconds of adult's model across 3 consecutive sessions, 2 settings, and 2 therapists.

Cognitive:

C:1:1 +2 During a structured activity with identical toys, pictures, or materials, Janie will match at least 5 pairs of objects or pictures, after following an adult model and direction to do so, with 2 adults and across 3 of 4 consecutive sessions.

Play:

P:1:7 When playing with toys and routine household objects, Janie will demonstrate use of a range of 8 objects in purposeful play on her own body, including actions such as donning a hat, combing or brushing hair, placing glasses on her head, sipping from a cup, talking on a phone across 2 or more people, at home and in therapy across 3 consecutive play sessions.

P:1:8 During structured play time, Janie will follow verbal directions to finish a simple close-ended task (shape sorter, simple puzzle), and when asked to "clean up" will place at least 2 pieces into container with no further prompt with parents and therapists at home for 3 consecutive sessions.

Fine Motor:

FM:1:6 Janie will demonstrate skill of putting together and taking apart pop beads, duplos, bristle blocks, or similar materials independently with 2 play partners for 3 consecutive days.

Gross Motor:

GM:1:1 Janie will kick, roll, or throw a large ball in any direction back and forth across 3 rounds with another person, with 2 play partners across 3 consecutive sessions.

Behavior:

B:1:2 Janie will sit in a chair, facing an adult, without difficulty for 1 to 2 minutes during structured, pleasurable sensory social or joint activity routines, 3 out of 4 opportunities with 2 different adults across 3 consecutive sessions.

ESDM is an integrative therapy, so skills are not worked toward discretely. Each activity typically encompasses a few goals at a time. For example, singing "If You're Happy and You Know It" encouraged Janie's eye contact, joint attention, and sensory stimulation.

Establishing Routines

Familiarity gave Janie comfort and security, so Megan immediately built up a few routines that she could expect in the sessions. Megan always greeted her with a big wave and "Hi, Janie!" In response, Janie would usually jump up and down, peek through Megan's bags of toys, or run into the sunroom to begin.

Megan recorded in her EI notes that "singing gains her attention," and she often started the sessions with songs that went along with books or finger plays, such as "Itsy-Bitsy Spider," "The Wheels on the Bus," and Janie's favorite, "Five

Little Monkeys." Janie especially liked Megan's *Five Little Ducks* book. Within a few weeks our entire family learned the words and sang it to her on demand. Songs invariably sparked interaction from Janie, such as dancing with Megan to the "Hokey Pokey" or holding hands for "Row Your Boat." Megan added to and varied activities to keep them dynamic for Janie and to prevent her from fixating on a set routine.

Since Janie rarely engaged in pretend play, Megan established routines around dolls, such as dressing and feeding. In those first few weeks, they also focused on cause/effect play routines, like stacking and crashing blocks and dropping cars down slides. Megan would hold a car at the top of the slide, look to Janie, and say, "Ready, set..." and soon Janie began shouting, "Go!"

Janie particularly liked when they painted with watercolors at the easel as she learned to follow the steps of dipping the brush in the water, dabbing the brush with paint, and painting on the paper. Bubbles were a staple in the sessions; they worked on discriminating size with big and small bubbles.

Megan and Janie put the toys away together as soon as they finished an activity. At the end of each session, Megan packed up her toys and said with a big smile and wave, "Bye, Janie!"

Social First, Talking Second

Megan told me early on she had no doubt Janie would speak in paragraphs by the time she started preschool. I could not imagine Janie saying more than a few words at a time and was surprised at this rare prediction from Megan. I was more surprised when she followed up by saying that talking was not a primary goal. She explained that Janie first needed to better understand the social nuances and contexts around speaking and communicating in general. Janie had the words, but she did not understand how to use them.

Working together at the easel one day, Janie identified each letter they drew and its sound for Megan. I asked her if we should start teaching Janie to read, as she seemed ready and interested. I also thought reading would give her confidence later on, especially since she struggled more than her peers in so many other areas.

"No," Megan was firm. She sat on the floor as Janie colored at the easel, and explained that Janie's memory and knowledge of the alphabet, numbers, and colors were a great strength. Rather than strengthening those strengths, we needed to focus on using her strengths to build up her deficits. Her advice made sense and I followed it, but selfishly I did want to teach Janie to read.

Learning to Communicate

Janie had very little understanding of communication. She knew many words, but not how to use them, verbally or nonverbally. Watching Megan draw communication out of Janie, particularly during those early weeks of therapy, was fascinating. I thought Janie completely non-responsive when we asked her questions. She did in fact have strong opinions, but did not know how to express them.

From the beginning of treatment, Megan would usually offer Janie two choices of what to play. She would hold up a doll and then a puzzle, for example, and say, "Would you like to play babies or do a puzzle?" The first time she did so, I told her that Janie would not answer. Megan nodded, but kept her eyes on Janie.

"Oh! You want to do a puzzle!"

I hopped off the couch to look at Janie. "She answered you?"

Megan explained that Janie did not need to vocalize what she wanted just yet. She could understand Janie's preference by which toy she looked at or reacted to in some way (such as showing excitement) when she held up one toy over another.

I asked Janie questions frequently, but had stopped expecting a response. I now realized she'd given me answers all along, and I had never picked up on them.

Megan often sat Janie in a little rocking chair directly in front of her, so that they interacted at eye level. She paused activities mid-stream to encourage communication from Janie, which might be jumping up and down to show she wanted Megan to blow more bubbles for instance. Janie started repeating words, gesturing, or using eye contact to keep an activity going. By the end of October, Megan noted that Janie was "reaching to choose from an array of two objects and consistently handing me toys to request help or start an activity."

Janie's imitation skills have been critical to her learning. In all types of activities, she copied Megan's actions. One day when they were at Janie's little table stamping, Megan asked if Janie was left-handed. She is right-handed, but mirrored Megan so exactly that she stamped with her left instead. Janie echoed single words and eventually phrases, memorizing the words that match the contexts. She did not always understand the words, just that they applied to a specific situation.

Janie gestured very little. She did not wave and had stopped pointing. Megan used dramatic gestures as she spoke to help Janie understand their meaning and to begin to use them herself.

Bubbles prompted a breakthrough in gesturing for Janie. Megan would blow a bubble and then say, "Clap!" as she clapped the bubble, or "Stomp!" as they stomped bubbles on the floor, or "Poke!" as she popped a bubble with her finger. Janie copied Megan verbally and physically. Soon after, she started pointing to express her preferences.

Janie also had trouble generalizing some words beyond a specific situation. For example, the word "up" in "pull up the shades" did not relate in Janie's mind to going "up" the stairs. We dramatically voiced certain words in different situations to help her understand that words could be used in more than one context.

Engage, Engage, Engage

Megan was Janie's therapist several hours a week, but our family members were her therapists around the clock. The more interaction with people the more Janie would come out of her own inner world and better understand the world around her.

We sang and danced with Janie, played instruments (beating drums and taking turns copying each other's beats, for example), rolled cars back and forth, pushed dolls in strollers around the house, played dress up, and pretended to have picnics and tea parties. We imitated Janie, and she imitated us. We joined into her solitary games. We yelled, "My turn!" and "Your turn!" to help her understand the reciprocity of play. When we read to Janie, we encouraged her to point to pictures and then reacted ("Oh! You like the rabbit!").

Megan also told me to model nonverbal gestures for Janie —nodding, shaking my head, and pointing. Instead of asking Janie to "Say 'outside'" when she screamed by the door, I would instead open the door while animatedly exclaiming, "Outside!" I constantly commented on whatever could be commented on, hoping she would catch on. Megan did not want Janie to simply ask questions, as natural conversations consist more of continuous comments than questions.

Comparing Objects

Janie loved to compare two similar objects—from magnetic letters on the refrigerator to a board book that matched a picture book. I found her sitting in her crib one day holding two Cookie Monster stuffed animals, staring from one to the other. She liked to set up a duo of toy laptops in the sunroom and go to work switching back and forth between them. She often toted similar toys around with her for extended periods of time.

I asked our EI supervisor, Ann Marie, if children on the spectrum typically carry objects around. She said that was common, often without a functional purpose, like carrying a DVD cover. But to me, this was not the same; comparing things fascinated Janie. She would focus on one object (such as mastering a toy computer game) or two similar objects for a few days and then lose interest, as if she was working to understand them and then tossing them aside once she felt she did.

One week Janie was fixated on a snake stuffed animal. She took the blue, four foot snake everywhere, even holding it throughout an entire ballet class. Megan had a difficult time conducting one of their sessions together since Janie would not let go of the snake. I had to hide it before Megan came the next day. Several days later, Janie forgot about the snake and moved on to another toy.

Megan was not overly concerned about her holding objects, which she thought gave Janie a sense of security and stability. She only stepped in when they prevented Janie from participating in activities because her hands were occupied. If Janie put the toys down to play something else, I quickly hid them, or Megan would have the toys watch Janie play, as she had with the giraffe and bear on the tiny couch. Janie sometimes tolerated letting go of the toys and sometimes not. Every so often she cried and became upset in these instances and in other activities, but usually only for a few minutes, as Megan would redirect her to a new activity.

Discipline

To my surprise, neither Ann Marie nor Megan thought time-outs were appropriate for Janie. Time-outs had been my go-to discipline method. Walking away from a temper tantrum was out too. Unlike my other kids, Janie could not understand consequences or how a time-out related to her behavior.

Instead, Megan stressed redirecting. If Janie colored on furniture, I told her "no" and pulled out a coloring book. When the rest of the kids and I were all set for a walk and Janie refused to join us, I enticed her into the stroller with Twizzlers. If she would not comply with a request, I never gave her a time-out or told her she had to do something. I cajoled her.

In Janie's mind, the world revolved around her, more so than with typical kids. If she would rather be doing something else, she refused dinner or a bath until I sweetened the offer. If I forced her to do anything, she shut down into full tantrum mode. She could not empathize that I had made her dinner or receptively understand that she needed to get clean in the tub. That would come in time.

I also could not raise my voice at Janie. Yelling at kids is obviously not good discipline, but I can lose my patience at times and it happens in our house. I do not yell at Janie though. Her stress is acute when I raise my voice at the other kids. Me being upset directly at her rocks her foundation.

Redirecting was exhausting, but necessary for Janie.

New Goals

By mid-October, Janie warmed up quickly to Megan when she arrived each morning—smiling, using more eye contact, and readily following her into activities. Megan noted that Janie was "tolerating my actions with minimal protest" and "pulls away less often" with hands-on interactions. She was ready for a new set of goals as well, having met most of the initial milestones.

In terms of receptive language (understanding what is said to her), Megan focused on Janie more consistently looking to an object pointed out to her; to "look, reach, smile, or gesture" when a familiar song played; and follow one-step, routine instructions paired with verbal cues (or hints). Janie started to follow simple directions, such as "Get it," "Push," "Put in," and "Clean up." Megan also incorporated a "Stop! Go!" running game into many of the sessions.

When Janie and I went for walks, I would say, "Janie, look!" and point to a bird or flower. She would attune her gaze to where I pointed (a new skill for her) and soon began pointing things out to me. Janie was also more often than not responding to her own name.

Expressively, Megan pushed Janie to ask for help by handing an object to someone, pointing to choose, and making eye contact. Janie began giving toys to Megan to initiate games, such as our tea set or pulling out Play-Doh from Megan's bag. Janie had more eye contact and gestures in their routines, particularly in the finger plays with songs.

Janie was also saying and signing the word "more." At meals for example, Megan had me serve Janie a small portion of her favorite foods, but keep most out of reach to encourage her to point or request "more."

Socially, Megan focused on Janie smiling at people, participating in familiar sensory social games, and turn taking. They also worked on fine and gross motor skills: putting together and pulling apart pop beads; drawing marks, lines, scribbles, and dots; and kicking, rolling, and throwing a ball with another person.

Megan set as a goal for Janie to imitate actions on objects, such as Play-Doh. She had shown little interest in Play-Doh previously because she had no idea how to play with it. Megan worked with Janie to press designs into Play-Doh and to poke, squish, and roll it. Although Janie at first did not like to touch Play-Doh and would point at Megan to poke it, she eventually became comfortable. In one session Megan noted, "She put it away, which means she needed to touch it. This was great."

Megan was methodically teaching Janie to better understand the world around her, and Janie was noticeably different. By November, Janie's tantrums subsided considerably. She consistently pointed to what she wanted and even responded to directions. One day she pointed to the front door and said, "Open, Dad." We all stopped in our tracks asking each other if we all heard her.

Janie was changing outside of the home too. She participated more in her classes, instead of relying on me to enable her engagement. At ballet one day, the teacher picked up each child to sashay around the room. The teacher and I were both stunned when Janie walked up to her and held up her arms for a turn.

Janie at Work

Although Janie was always happy when Megan arrived and seemed to enjoy most of their activities, Megan explained that therapy was actually hard work for Janie. Engaging with another person for sustained amounts of time and often in unfamiliar activities did not come naturally for her. While Megan did not encourage Janie's predilection for her preschool computers and interactive toys, she recognized that they relaxed Janie and gave her pleasure, so used them as breaks for her in therapy. Janie's treatment was delivered through play, but she had to work hard while she played hard.

6

SPEECH THERAPY

About two months into ESDM therapy with Megan, speech therapy came into the mix. Janie's Early Intervention language pathologist, Abby, showed up at our house for the first session in late November. She carried a large L.L. Bean tote brewing with toys. Thirtyish, Abby had long black hair, usually tied up into a pony tail while she worked, a tiny nose ring (that Luke pointed out), and like Megan, a huge smile.

Janie played in the sunroom while we talked, and I explained her reticence around new people. Abby engaged with Janie in a friendly way, but minimally until Janie came to her—a technique everyone from Early Intervention seemed to have mastered. She listened closely and took notes while I told her about Janie. She wrote in her EI report that first day, "Janie will label things, jargons [using unintelligible language] while playing, and sings many songs, but she is not yet using her language to communicate."

Janie wandered over to us when Abby set up several wind-up toys in a row on the floor. She sat next to Abby when she pulled out her iPad, pointing at it and smiling at her.

When Abby returned the following week for their second session, Janie warmed up quickly and worked with her for 45 minutes straight, only leaving her seat when Abby began writing her EI note. Abby typically sat on the floor at the edge of our sectional couch with her tote bag beside her. She had Janie sit in a child-sized chair directly in front of her, so their eye contact was level.

Knowing Janie's affinity for music, Abby pulled out a small xylophone, encouraging Janie to say "up," "down," and "tap." She put her hand on her chest and then guided Janie's hand to her own chest while saying "me," demonstrating how to indicate that she would like a turn.

By this time, Janie's echolalia was peaking. She repeated "up," "down," "tap," "me," and just about everything else that came out of Abby's mouth. Echolalia (the automatic repetition of vocalizations) is a common symptom of autism. I had heard Janie echo people plenty of times before, but never to the extent she imitated Abby. A sinking feeling came over me as I listened to her parroting Abby.

At the end of the hour, Abby made an observation about the echolalia: Janie did not repeat requests or praise; she echoed what she did not understand. In other words, Janie was not mimicking simply to mimic; she struggled to make sense of what was going on around her. Just like memorizing, repeating was a tactic to help her understand. The cloud lifted a bit.

Abby's bag was also filled with dozens of puzzles and books, plastic bugs that pop together, and a few other toys. Although the toys rarely varied, there were enough choices that Janie always came right over to pick something out. Abby kept puzzle pieces together in plastic bags that she opened with a "Ziiiip!" She would hold the bag up and wait for Janie to say "me" with the appropriate sign of her hand to her chest before passing her each piece. They read books together too, Janie pointing to or labeling the pictures that Abby asked her about.

In December, when Janie was nearly two and half years old, she began using words to communicate. Abby noted that Janie was spontaneously saying "mine," "hot," and "tap" and labeling a few animals without prompting. Abby would ask her, "What does a cow say?" and Janie could answer "moo" or the appropriate sounds for different animals. She pointed and signed "me" when Abby offered her the choice of two activities. The echolalia decreased with each session as Janie began to understand their routine together.

Megan worked with Janie in the mornings while Sarah and Luke were at school. Abby squeezed us into a slot on Monday afternoons when the older kids were home. I tried to shoo Sarah and Luke upstairs when Abby arrived, but Janie always followed them up. They begged to watch, so I usually set them up with their homework at the island in our kitchen, while I nursed or held Finn on the couch watching Janie and Abby. Within minutes, Sarah and Luke would drift over, lounging behind me with their elbows perched on the back of the sectional. By spring, they took front row seats on the couch watching entire sessions, Janie's own peanut gallery, chuckling whenever she made funny comments or got confused.

Speech therapy chugged along smoothly with Janie consistently making gains from week to week.

7

AUTISM AND THE SENSES

Running, Jumping, Squeezing

Janie is a runner and a jumper. She could run as long and as far as Sarah and Luke, albeit at a slower pace. She often took off on a path by our house that circles the neighborhood, only turning back to smile and laugh when we would yell for her to stop. She constantly jumped on the couches and beds.

If knocked down in the crossfire of a pillow fight, Janie would giggle as she pulled herself up again. I sometimes piled the three kids on my bed to bomb them with pillows. Sarah and Luke liked to guard Janie, repelling as many of the incoming pillows as they could as she blissfully jumped away behind them, never minding if she got hit. I attributed her pillow-bashing passion to her wild side, not realizing there might be more to it.

After their first few sessions, Megan asked me about Janie's jumping on the couch as well as her tendency to bend down and put her head on the floor between her feet. Megan showed up the next morning with bright, thin, square-shaped pillows. She made up games jumping from pillow to pillow, Janie following along like a duckling.

Megan laid Janie down on a few of the pillows, while pushing another pillow softly and quietly on her chest, tummy, then legs. She lay motionless throughout until Megan stopped. Then Janie handed the pillow back for Megan to do it again.

Megan also squeezed Janie's arms and legs with her hands, slowly moving down her limbs, then shaking them out, saying, "Squeeze, squeeze, squeeze! Wiggle, wiggle!" Janie always signed for "more."

Janie craved physical sensory stimulation when she was over- or under-stimulated. When she became overexcited or upset, we squeezed her until she calmed down. Megan recommended regulating her sensory seeking tendencies through music and movement as well.

As I began to understand the connection between Janie's autism and her sensory sensitivities, I thought often of the "squeeze machine" Temple Grandin built to deliver the pressure that soothed her. Grandin was diagnosed with autism when she was a child, at a time when very little was known about the disorder and much of it misperceived. Her doctor recommended she be institutionalized. Her mother disagreed and pushed Grandin to learn to speak, which she finally did at age four, and helped teach her how to interact socially.

Grandin went on to earn a Ph.D. and become one of the world's leading designers of livestock-handling facilities, due to her ability to think in vivid detail and understand animals so uniquely. She has written several books and lectures worldwide about autism and also the cattle industry. What I find most impressive about Grandin is that she was the first person with autism to articulate and explain the disorder so thoroughly from a first-hand perspective.

While I admire Temple Grandin immensely, I felt some heartache recognizing this aspect of autism in my daughter. In the end, pressure made Janie feel good. It is what it is.

Megan also noticed that Janie refused to hold hands with anyone outside our family. Megan routinely laid out her "squishing" pillows, and together they stepped on them like lily pads while singing "Ring Around the Rosie." Janie loved the song, but only minimally tolerated Megan holding her hand. So Megan had her hold a doll's hand between them or I would join in. After a few months, Janie became comfortable holding Megan's hand, and the handholding aversion faded.

Occupational Therapy Evaluation

Megan set up an occupational therapy (OT) evaluation through Early Intervention to see if Janie needed OT services. She wanted the occupational therapist's input on regulatory strategies for Janie's jumping, her reluctance to touch other people's hands, and her tendency to chew on toothbrushes.

The EI occupational therapist, Kelly, came to our house with Ann Marie in November to observe one of Megan's sessions and evaluate Janie. Her brown hair loose and wavy, Kelly dressed in a long, baggy shirt and leggings. Her eyes twinkled like a grandmother's as she watched and played with children. Her mouth was usually fixed in a soft smile.

Kelly hung back initially to avoid making Janie anxious. Like most EI therapists, she first pointed out all of Janie's strengths and then made useful recommendations. Off the bat, she noticed Janie's low average muscle tone. She explained that standing still for a period of time would be difficult for Janie. She recommended using vertical planes, such as working at the easel or putting Colorforms on the windows, so Janie could bend down and stand up for fine motor and vertical stimulation.

She agreed with Megan that Janie sought sensory input to help regulate herself—jumping, running, squishing from pillows, squeezing, pressure on the top of her head, and climbing. I should offer those activities when she needed that type of arousal. Kelly suggested other movement activities as well, such as push and ride-on toys, and especially outdoor play on the swings and slide. To add a social element, she encouraged me to play "Stop! Go!" games within the sensory activity. If Janie initiated a play action, she wanted me to expand on it, either adding an idea or lengthening a game by saying, "One more time!"

With Janie's tendency to carry toys and other objects around with her, Kelly stressed emptying her hands as much as possible. She recommended an electric toothbrush for all the chewing, but Janie was afraid of them at that point (as well as remote control cars and ball popper toys). Kelly encouraged us to keep up Megan's handholding strategies as well.

I have been asked many times throughout evaluations and different therapy sessions about Janie's reaction to touching sand, washing her hands, or eating particular foods. The feel of certain textures bothers many children on the spectrum.

Megan sometimes put lotion on Janie's hands and legs to gauge her comfort. Janie loved it, especially when she squished the lotion herself. They played with sand and washed their hands together. On Megan's advice, we filled her water table with uncooked rice to scoop and sift. Janie fortunately was fine with it all. She was picky with food, but more about taste and unfamiliarity than feel. Although Janie was comfortable with most textures, Kelly did not want her to backtrack. She also suggested filling a box with uncooked beans and hidden toys to find.

Janie had limited sensory issues, aside from craving pressure, which was easy to recognize and deliver to her. Kelly did not think Janie's sensory seeking tendencies were significant enough to warrant OT. Megan and I recorded all of Kelly's advice and incorporated it into her sessions and daily life.

8

SPARKING IMAGINARY PLAY

The most dramatic transformation I saw in Janie was with her pretend play. ESDM therapy essentially turned on her imagination.

Megan pointed out that Janie did not know how to play with many of her toys. Most children will naturally mash, poke, and pull apart Play-Doh without being shown how. I remember putting a few slabs of Play-Doh in front of Janie while I cooked dinner one evening and was surprised to see her look it over, then walk away without even touching it. She so often veered for electronic games because they require no imagining or creativity, just pushing buttons, watching lights, and listening to sounds.

Janie did not intuitively know how to play with many toys, but she used her imitation skills to learn. Once shown how to play with a toy, she would copy, and over time that imitation turned into understanding.

Megan and Janie logged many hours with Play-Doh during therapy sessions. They first focused on Janie becoming comfortable touching and manipulating it—poking, rolling, making balls, stamping, and eventually moving onto forming shapes and people. Megan would then turn their Play-Doh creations into stories, of yellow ducks on a blue pond for example.

Prior to therapy, Janie had shown very little interest in dolls. So Megan and Janie spent countless hours playing baby dolls together. They would feed, dress, and change the dolls, and rock them to sleep. Simple play became more elaborate over time, as they added in a bath routine and pushing their "babies" in strollers. Janie mirrored Megan, happily following along in the sequences and absorbing. As the months passed, Janie began to offer suggestions and make up scenarios herself, such as cooking soup for the dolls. Tea parties were a big hit with Janie, especially setting up a cup and plate for each doll and serving her guests. Christopher, Sarah, Luke, and I were knee deep in dolls and tea parties for months.

As Janie caught onto pretend play and learned to use her own imagination, Megan expanded the play with other toys as well. They built houses out of blocks and made little families of toy animals who might be expecting company or going on a car trip. They set up elaborate train tracks throughout our sunroom and played with cars and trains on the tracks. Megan and Janie sat side by side on rocking horses, going on journeys and stopping to feed the horses.

By spring, Janie often skipped her afternoon nap and instead filled that time playing with her princess dolls. She created storylines and even different voices for the characters. Engrossed in her imagination, she could play princesses for an hour or two straight.

We have leaned on her love of pretend play to ease her rigidity in other areas. Janie has become more and more particular about what she eats and often would rather not eat at all. So we started animating her meals—her steak begs her not to eat it, her vegetables hide under her bread so she will *never* find them, or her chicken is sassy. Then we ask Janie what she is going to do about her mischievous food. If we come up with a good storyline, she will clear the plate. Luke and Sarah are masters at getting her to eat.

Janie's imagination now runs wild, and it's wonderful.

9

SIBLING SESSIONS

Janie with Sarah and Luke

From early on, Janie preferred Luke to Sarah—and Sarah noticed. Whenever Luke tackled Janie to the floor, she hopped back up and chased him down for more. When Sarah pulled her into a hug, Janie squirmed out of her grasp. Luke's antics were hilarious to Janie, while Sarah's attempts to play with her sister were often rebuffed. When Sarah did come across an activity that drew Janie in, like singing Lady Gaga together, she would not let Luke join in or even play it on his own with Janie.

Sarah came to me upset more than a few times. I encouraged her to find common ground with Janie, namely her little sister's toys and games. Sarah's time would come; soon Janie would be into all sorts of girly stuff that held no interest for Luke. An "in the future" solution was little consolation to Sarah. I asked Megan for advice.

Megan explained that it was sometimes easier for girls with autism to engage with boys rather than other girls based on the nature of the activities. Boys tend to participate in activities involving motor skills (chase, climbing, building things), whereas girls often veer towards dramatic or pretend play with detailed themes that involve frequent verbal communication and attention to nonverbal cuing, as well as fine motor activities, such as art. Some girls with autism find better success playing with their male peers; they can more easily understand playing chase or active games that require less sustained attention and less emphasis on reciprocal communication.

I relayed Megan's insights to Sarah, who for an eight-year-old, understood surprisingly well. She adjusted her play, and Janie was hooked almost immediately. As her pretend play in particular expanded her interests, Janie sought out Sarah as much as Luke. No one can make her laugh like Luke, but when Sarah pulls out her American Girl dolls or sets up a mermaid adventure, Janie sticks to her sister like a barnacle.

First Family Session

Sarah and Luke asked about Megan constantly. They were curious about this person who played such a central role in Janie's life. When school let out for Christmas break, they finally met her. Megan structured a session around Sarah and Luke, focusing on ways they should play with Janie (who lapped the couch in excitement when she realized her siblings would join in that day).

They began by playing "Ring Around the Rosie," Megan instructing Sarah and Luke to hold Janie's hands while they circled in slow and fast motion, then freezing when she yelled, "Stop!" Next came "Duck, Duck, Goose," with one sibling helping Janie take a turn as the "ducker" until she understood the game. They also played chase with the "it" person carrying a small towel, so that Janie could get the concept of playing tag.

Then they all sat down at Janie's small table with Play-Doh. Megan had Sarah and Luke offer their sister a choice of colors and model rolling, pushing, poking, and cutting the Play-Doh. They put the Play-Doh lids tightly on the cans to keep Janie from holding them in her hands while she worked.

Next, Sarah and Luke took turns kicking a soccer ball back and forth with Janie.

Megan told the kids what she told me, to give Janie single word choices and opportunities to point or shake her head "yes" or "no" while they played. They followed her directions with military precision and from then on approached their play with Janie as Megan had instructed them.

More Therapy with Sarah and Luke

Anxiously anticipating another session with Megan, Sarah and Luke got their chance several weeks later over the February break. Megan began the session with Barbie dolls, coaching Sarah to offer Janie choices of a few dolls and outfits, and to follow sequences of play, such as sleeping, waking, feeding, sitting on the couch, or riding in a car. When Janie moved on to her mermaid dolls, Megan asked Sarah to present Janie with two mermaids to choose from, then lead her into broader pretend play.

Luke joined in for music play. Megan told them to sing Janie songs she knew and to take turns picking the song. As the four of them danced to the iPod, Megan encouraged the kids to copy Janie's actions and for her to copy theirs. To keep Janie's attention, she had them intermittently yell "Stop!" "Freeze!" "Go!" "Watch me!" and "Janie look!" Next, they played dress-up in front of a mirror, letting Janie pick out shoes, hats, gloves, and jewelry.

Megan then set up their last activity, an obstacle course. The three kids began by crawling through a tunnel, then jumped onto beanbags, hopped on Twister spots and over scattered toys, climbed overturned child-sized armchairs, and then started the course again. Megan had Luke go first, gently restraining Janie with a hand to her chest. When she finally said, "Your turn!" Janie was off and running with Sarah trailing behind her.

Janie tackled the obstacle course while Sarah and Luke

helped her along wherever she needed it. Once they finished the loop and reached the beginning again, Janie would dart in front of Luke to head into the tunnel. Megan could catch her practically in mid-air. She would tell her that it was Luke's turn, and she would be next.

"It's okay, she can go ahead of me," Luke said to Megan nearly every time around.

"You go Luke," Megan told him. "Janie will go after you."

Megan held Janie back like a miniature bull until Luke had crawled halfway through the tunnel. Then she would yell, "Your turn, Janie!" and she was off again.

They did the obstacle course fast and furious for about 15 minutes. Each time they started over, Janie pushed past Luke, who stepped aside for her until Megan intervened and had Janie wait her turn.

Afterwards we all sat on the couch, and Megan told the kids how well they did. She asked Luke if he understood why she would not let Janie go ahead of him. He shook his head.

Megan spent about ten minutes explaining how Janie is learning to take turns. She talked about ballet class, where Janie cuts to the front anytime they form a line. Learning how to take turns would help her in playing with kids her age. The purpose of the obstacle course was teaching Janie to wait her turn. When Megan finished, she asked them, "Do you have questions about anything else we did today?"

Luke raised his hand. "Why couldn't I just let Janie go in front of me?"

I laughed and howled at Luke. Megan said, "That's a good question," and explained it all again.

Megan told me that Janie's siblings would be her best therapists, and she was right. The kids set up obstacle courses and played chase, "Duck, Duck, Goose," and Play-Doh like they were getting paid for it. They often took on Megan's tone when talking to Janie. They were truly mini-therapists. I was surprised not only by their dedication to their sister, but also their capacity to understand her struggles and needs.

PART III

JANIE'S STEPS OUT OF AUTISM (JANIE FROM 2½ – 3 YEARS OLD)

10

PROGRESS AND REGRESSION

New Goals

Janie continued progressing well through December. She and Megan had an easy rapport. Megan knew what to target and exactly how hard to push, and Janie responded. She reached her next set of ESDM goals.

I asked Megan if Janie would still have the PDD-NOS diagnosis once she achieved the final set of goals. I saw a flash of empathy in her expression before she cleared it and explained that achieving these goals would not erase the diagnosis. Regardless, Janie was ready for her third set of goals within three months. Megan laid out her next milestones:

1. *Following one step directions*
2. *Pointing to pictures of objects or family members*
3. *Retrieving objects when told, "Get x"*
4. *Using signs, gestures, or words to make requests, say all done, help, or protest*
5. *Using at least 20 names to request activities or objects*
6. *Shaking and nodding her head*
7. *Showing objects when requested ("Show me x")*

8. *Spontaneously pointing to interesting objects to share experiences*
9. *Responding to hi/bye with wave and words*
10. *Playing chase*
11. *Sorting objects into like groups*
12. *Searching for missing pieces*
13. *Taking turns with simple action toys (gives and takes back)*
14. *Combining play themes with dolls*
15. *Imitating five or more actions on Play-Doh*
16. *Imitating strokes with crayon or marker*
17. *Stringing beads*
18. *Kicking a ball to a target*
19. *Removing two items of clothing*
20. *Jumping over an object*

In light of these new objectives, I asked Megan what to get Janie for Christmas. She stressed pretend play toys, particularly dolls that do not make noise (no toys in general that make sounds and light up) and two matching sets of doll accessories (two bottles, two spoons, two diapers)—one set for Janie and one for Megan or another playmate.

Some Words and Gestures

By December, Janie consistently pointed to communicate what she wanted or to share an experience. Megan asked me to put a favorite toy in a Tupperware container up on the mantel. Janie pointed to request the toy and sometimes labeled it, although not yet with coordinated eye contact.

She had a few spontaneous words, such as "mine" (also to request) and "my turn." Janie began initiating activities, saying "patty-feet" or "peek-a-boo" to get a game going for example. Megan continued to push the social side of communication (looking to people, gesturing, and sharing experiences) over actual words.

We focused next on "yes" and "no" along with shaking and nodding her head, since they were not coming naturally for Janie. Megan would present Janie with two toys, finger puppets for example, offering her the less desirable one first so that she would have to push it away or shake her head no. We modeled headshakes and nods constantly. She began to shake her head no in December. The occasional head nod followed a few weeks later.

Waving (which most children do by age one) had not appeared yet for Janie either. When Megan arrived or left, she waved, I waved, and then I stood behind Janie and waved her hand for her. Janie started to wave on her own sporadically soon thereafter.

Janie called no one by name, except herself when she looked in the mirror and said, "Hi Janie." Megan put together a small photo album of our immediate family members and grandparents. We frequently asked Janie to name everyone.

Therapy Stamina

Janie began to tolerate more interruption of her preferred activities, particularly with her computer games, which she sought out less and less. She stuck with structured activities for longer periods of time. Janie sometimes became upset, but usually recovered in less than a minute without needing my reassurance, as she was easily redirected by Megan.

When Janie ran circles around the couch or struggled to focus on a task, Megan addressed her sensory seeking behavior in a variety of ways—pulling out our tricycle, throwing a ball through a hoop together, playing "Ring Around the Rosie," or singing songs with finger movements, like "Head, Shoulders, Knees, and Toes." Alternately, Megan would simply run around the house with Janie, calling out "Stop!" "Go!" "Fast!" and "Slow!" to encourage her to follow directions and share the experience.

. . .

Stranger Anxiety

A graduate student contacted Early Intervention to see if she could observe an ESDM session. Megan asked me more than once if I felt comfortable with the student coming. I didn't see why not.

Megan and Janie were playing Play-Doh when the student arrived. I pulled up a chair for her to watch, a couple feet back from the little table. Janie averted her gaze and put down the Play-Doh. Megan picked up on her anxiety quickly and asked the student to move farther back. The entire session was thrown off as Janie avoided eye contact and withdrew from their activities. With all of her progress, I had not anticipated that an unfamiliar person could cause Janie such intense discomfort.

Regression

Over the Christmas break, we did not have therapy sessions with Megan or Abby. Janie was sick after the holiday, so her sessions were cancelled the following week as well. I saw months of progress erased in days. Janie regressed in her behavior, play, and communication skills. Her sensory seeking tendencies became much more pronounced. She was running, jumping, and climbing all over the house. Megan suggested music and movement to help her regulate.

When Janie was healthy again, Abby came for a speech session. While reading a book together, she instructed Janie to say, "turn" when she finished a page. Whether she understood the direction or not, Janie wouldn't say "turn." She became increasingly upset as Abby refused to flip the pages and kept repeating, "turn…turn…turn…" to prompt Janie to follow suit.

Janie's frustration intensified until she finally retreated into the sunroom to find another book so that she could turn the pages herself. Abby followed her in and pressed on with "turn." I was nursing Finn on the couch, debating whether to step in. When Abby tried to pick her up to bring her back into the living room, Janie became hysterical.

Abby insisted that Janie was ready to communicate verbally, but I was not so sure. I relayed my concerns to Megan and Ann Marie about Abby understanding Janie well enough to realize that she had been pushed too far.

I was beside myself at the erosion of Janie's skills. Megan saw Janie's regression first-hand, with her extremely low frustration tolerance, sensory seeking behavior, and tears during their sessions.

Megan was concerned, but also explained that many children on the spectrum regress with an illness. She expected Janie to recover her skills in about the same amount of time she was sick (one week). Megan later confided to me that she had never seen a child with autism lose skills so drastically with an illness.

Janie not only recovered her skills, she took off.

11

CHATTY JANIE

After the excitement of Christmas passed and the older kids were back in school, Janie, Finn, and I went into what felt like hibernation for the long New England winter. Too cold for walks or playing outside, we were fairly homebound aside from Janie's music and ballet classes, Sarah and Luke's after school activities, and errands. Even playdates were tricky to arrange between Janie's morning therapy sessions and afternoon naps. We squeezed playdates in whenever we could to help with her social skills, but she still showed little interest in her peers. I went out with friends often to keep from going too stir-crazy.

Christopher was working and traveling quite a bit, but devoted most of his free time to the kids and me. He read Megan's notes each evening, and I kept him up on the skills we should target with Janie. Christopher worked from home a few times a month to watch Megan's sessions.

Sarah and Luke often asked what Janie did with Megan while they were at school—and when they could get in on another session. They continued to play with Janie exactly as Megan showed them. They read stories to her before bed if I was putting Finn to sleep, and when Sarah practiced violin, Janie planted herself right next to her sister to listen.

Once school was out in the afternoon, the house could get wild with kids. Janie trailed along whenever Sarah and Luke had friends over. A girlfriend of mine burst out laughing when she came in one day and saw a herd of kids in the sunroom crowded around Finn, perched up on a beanbag like a king on his throne. That sometime chaos and exposure to so many kids, in addition to all the one-on-one time with Sarah and Luke, gave Janie the opportunity to soak in social skills, many that only other kids can impart.

Old MacDonald

Janie had a few words when she began therapy, but she did not talk to communicate. As scary as the regression just after Christmas had been, as soon as Janie came out of it she launched to the next level with her social and communication skills. The first breakthrough came one day in January when Megan was singing "Old MacDonald." She paused after "and on that farm, he had a..." and held up a toy cow, sheep, or horse, waiting for Janie to say the name of the animal before she continued. Although Janie knew what a cow was and could say the word "cow," she struggled.

Finally, a high-pitched, "Cow!" squeaked out of her.

I was blown away that something so simple could be so challenging for Janie and also by her tenacity to succeed. I could see the tension in her body as she focused her whole being on that cow. Megan kept the song going, drawing forth from Janie the names of all sorts of barn animals in a voice I had never heard her use.

Megan called it "pressured speech," contorted from all the effort getting it out. "Old MacDonald" turned the page on a new chapter for Janie.

Food as the Carrot

At lunch one day soon after the "cow" breakthrough, Janie

was eating at our kitchen island and spotted an open bag of popcorn on the counter. She may have pointed to it, but I had my back to her, loading the dishwasher. I turned around when Janie became frustrated. I could not understand why she was agitated, until she blurted out, "Popcorn!"

"Popcorn" was the first word she used to verbally indicate what she wanted without prompting. It came out pressured but discernible. I piled her tray with popcorn as soon as she said it. Abby had recently remarked that frustration was a great incentive for Janie to encourage her to speak.

Megan immediately seized on the "popcorn" coup and incorporated Janie's lunchtime into her sessions. We continued to offer Janie choices at meals, but instead of simply pointing, we prompted her to say what she wanted. I would hold up bread and say, "Bread. B-b-bread," and wait for her to say "bread" or simply the "b" sound before handing it to her. Janie was game, saying the first sound and often the entire word, such as "nut" and even "peanut butter."

Soon she asked for food not presented to her, like pizza and cheese. She used a combination of pointing, gesturing, and saying or signing "for me" (which she had learned from Abby) to request food. Megan suggested I eat with Janie so that her meals were more social.

Open!

We routinely put one of Janie's favorite toys into a Tupperware container with a tight lid, but instead of placing it out of her reach, we now left the container at her level, so that she would have to say "open" to get the toy. When they pulled out Play-Doh, Megan would pause with a can in her hand until Janie said, "Open!" After some modeling, Janie quickly caught on and generalized "open" across different types of situations.

"Open" became such a powerful word for Janie that she often *over*generalized it. Getting into the car one day, Janie tried to reach for my sunglasses up by the rear view mirror. She finally gave up and yelled, "Open!" So we focused next on "help" and offering the appropriate words when she fell back on "open" for requests.

Narrating Her Play

I never imagined a child narrating their playtime like a sports commentator, but that is exactly what Megan taught Janie to do. I took her to a playspace one day and watched as she moved from the trampoline to the balls to the slide giving everyone within earshot a blow by blow, calling out, "Jump! Throw! Bounce! Slide!"

Megan stressed that most conversations are not full of questions, but more comments layered upon comments between people. She did not want Janie simply asking questions to interact with others, but to have more natural conversations. Megan noted that Janie was "commenting on most actions that happen with rote phrases and spontaneous single words and gestures."

Janie memorized and matched phrases to situations. When she played ball with Megan, she would call out, "I got it!" "There it is!" and "Over there!" as well as spontaneous words like "Oops!" and "Wow!" Instead of screaming by the back door, she started saying, "Show me outside!"

Two Words Together

In addition to her memorized phrases, Janie began putting two words together on her own to make requests and show interest. At lunch one day she said, "Cheese for me." She consistently signed and said, "More," "All done," and also "My turn" while patting her chest.

Megan noted, "Many new words that Janie used previously to label pictures are now being used to communicate preferences." When Janie offered a verbal comment or request, Megan always followed her lead to reinforce her efforts to communicate.

Within a few weeks, "Jump!" became "I jump!" Megan then encouraged us to model "-ing" words to narrate her actions. Janie quickly progressed from "Run!" to "I run!" to "I running!"

Janie said her first unprompted "yes" with Christopher, and we all cheered. By the end of January, she answered questions consistently with "yes" or "no" and the accompanying nod or shake of her head (although nodding, even two years later, is still a bit stilted for Janie).

Speech Therapy

Although she could have pushed Janie more gently, Abby realized before Megan and I that she was ready to advance to the next level from a communication standpoint. After the "turn" session ended with Janie in hysterics, I dreaded her reaction to Abby's subsequent visit. Apparently, it was water under the bridge. Janie ran to the door to greet Abby and happily attended to her for the next 45 minutes.

Abby noted that Janie was starting to express her preferences verbally in their sessions too. Like Megan, Abby stressed continuing to offer Janie choices to encourage her requesting. Janie said "Zip!" when she wanted to open Abby's bag of toys. She asked for songs on the xylophone by saying "twinkle" or "spider" for "Twinkle, Twinkle Little Star" and "The Itsy-Bitsy Spider" (Abby could play just about any tune). For the first time, Janie sang along with Abby.

Janie started naming toys she wanted to play with next. Abby pulled out her iPad more often, which Janie loved, particularly a vocabulary application that showed four pictures and asked, "Where is the chicken?" for example. Later along that winter, Janie greeted Abby one day with, "Play Abby iPad."

She commented with Abby too, such as "Going fast," "Big bubble," and "You get lion." Abby noted, "Janie used her language across activities and settings, generalizing her skills." Janie was tracking their play visually (using consistent eye contact) and articulating well.

Abby also observed that Janie's echolalia (repeating other people's words) continued to decrease. It seemed to come out only around new language and longer sentences that were more difficult for her to comprehend. Abby worked in tandem with Megan, each observing a session of the other's, so they could coordinate their approaches.

Counting Janie's Words

Janie's communication skills progressed full steam ahead into February. She referred to herself as both "Janie" and "I." She shared affect with others and made requests by pointing and with words. She also called Megan by her name for the first time.

Janie waved to and greeted her toys, although not yet people. Megan instructed me to fill in language for Janie. For example, when she climbed into my lap, I would say, "Oh, you want up!" She also had me work on "showing" behavior, such as pulling a toy out of a bag and saying, "Look Janie!" and then offering her a turn. When Janie echoed speech, Megan told us to knock a sentence down to simple words so that she could more easily understand it.

While most of her sentences at this point were memorized, Janie was starting to more naturally put words together in longer and longer strings. She was consistently coming out with two- and three-word spontaneous phrases, and up to four-word rote (memorized) phrases. She also directed her talking to others. Some of her breakthrough sentences in therapy with Megan were: "I have a yellow car," "We have big bubbles," "I want the red monkey," "I make a cut," "I'm thinking of the goose," and "You hug your dolly." She asked Abby one day, "How about the orange block?" I found myself constantly counting the words coming out of her mouth.

12

SIX MONTHS IN

Seismic shifts were taking place inside of Janie. I saw first-hand how much could hardwire between two and three years of age. During those initial six months of therapy, Megan led the way in reconnecting many of those wires before they became ingrained and possibly permanent symptoms of autism.

While Janie could not yet hold a sustained conversation or comprehend abstract concepts, she was now a whirlwind of words. Her communication deficits were shrinking markedly not only with her talking, but also with social aspects of communication, such as eye contact, joint attention, and sharing experiences with others.

Her social skills were also on a steep upward trajectory. Beginning to understand the give and take of relationships and play, Janie was eager to learn and caught on quickly. I started to notice a difference in Janie with other children as well. Six months into therapy, she joined an Early Intervention playgroup that helped ramp up her social skills. At this point, she was still uncomfortable around unfamiliar adults, but putting her toe in the water interacting with peers, like holding hands with girls at ballet class when they skipped across the room.

Janie's sensory issues and repetitive behaviors were sometimes present, particularly when she was sick, but usually minimal and easy to address.

We met with Dr. Shaw in April for our six-month check-in. She did not formally evaluate Janie again, but interacted with her for about half an hour. Dr. Shaw was happy with Janie's progress since her diagnosis, especially on the social side. Like Megan, she was less concerned with Janie talking and much more with gaining social skills.

Play Routines

Janie still smiled and jumped in excitement just about every time Megan arrived. By March, her ESDM goals centered on expanding her pretend play, with particular focus on her flexibility in adapting to change and new situations. Megan continually introduced new play routines to encourage shared social experiences, such as dancing together to the "Hokey Pokey" or hiding a toy under a cup for Janie to find. If she guessed correctly, they both cheered. When Megan pulled out a toy car that zoomed around the room, Janie happily raced after it yelling, "There it is!"

Megan and Janie played pretend with dolls and other toys, such as animal figures living in a house they built from blocks or Dora and her friends going on a car trip. So that Janie could better understand the concept of sharing, they also worked on "trading toys." They practiced saying "My turn" and "Your turn" during activities, such as piecing together a puzzle.

They continued with book routines and finger plays (Janie's favorite was "Five Green and Speckled Frogs"). She consistently interacted with Megan with shared eye contact and affect.

Pronouns, W Words, and Directions

Six months in, Janie narrated her play and regularly made comments in three- to five-word phrases, some memorized and some spontaneous, and the phrases were getting longer. One goal we focused on heavily in March and throughout the spring was increasing her use of names and pronouns. By this time, she addressed everyone in the family and Megan by name, but struggled distinguishing between "I," "me," "you," "mine," and "yours." Megan modeled pronouns while they dressed up in front of the mirror to help her better understand the distinctions.

We also asked her more "w" questions, like "Who wants the 'Wheels on the Bus'?" or "Where did the car go?" She could answer with "Me!" or "It's over there!"

Janie followed most of the one-step directions Megan gave her, such as pointing to a part of the body or a picture in a book, kicking or throwing a ball, sitting and standing, and putting toys away. She was ready to move on to two-step directions. Megan would ask her to retrieve an object and bring it to a specific person; for example, "Get the ball, and show it to Sarah." Janie responded and often showed Megan objects unprompted.

"Hullabaloo"

Puzzles, Play-Doh, music, books, bubbles, and balls were all constants of therapy. As described earlier, ESDM is an integrative therapy, so most of the activities Megan and Janie played together targeted more than one skill. A great example of an integrative game that Megan introduced to Janie around this time was "Hullabaloo."

"Hullabaloo" involves mats, music, and following directions. Megan spread out about a dozen colored mats on the floor, each with an image of an animal, food, or instrument. Music plays while the "Hullabaloo" voice instructs players to touch a color or animal, for instance, and move in a certain way. After a few turns, the player standing on a specific mat is announced the winner.

When told to "Hop over to a green pad," Janie would hop or find the correct mat, but usually not both. Over time, she learned to follow both sets of directions. Extremely engaged in the game, especially the music, she reveled in being the winner (particularly when the winner was told to "Take a bow" or "Do a funky dance"). We bought the game to keep up the therapy it provided.

Motor Skills

Megan and Janie often worked at the easel with stamps or drawing figures with markers. By March, Janie began drawing the eyes, nose, and mouth on faces and spontaneously added in a body for the first time. She could draw most of a person a few weeks later. They created faces with Play-Doh too.

Together they focused on a variety of gross motor skills in the spring: jumping, hopping on one foot, running and stopping, and tossing bean bags into a bucket or at targets. They threw and kicked balls to each other, practicing turn-taking and saying "mine" and "yours."

Family Therapy

After several months of therapy, Janie was a much more engaged member of our family. She retreated less into her own world, and when she did, we now had the skills to pull her back into ours.

Janie loved to play dolls with Sarah, and by this point often referred to her as "my Sarah." She sought out Luke for wrestling and running around the house. She milled around the iPod asking whomever was nearby, "Wanna dance?" She always ran to the door to greet Christopher when he came home from work.

By spring Megan had integrated Finn into the family therapy sessions too, helping Janie respond to and include him in play. Megan and Janie often sang to Finn, with the kids positioned across from each other so that Janie could look directly at him. They would also roll a ball back and forth with him.

When Finn moved into Janie's space and upset her, Megan prompted Janie with "My turn, Finn," or "No, Finn." Janie worked on allowing Finn to play with her toys, even if his turn only lasted a few seconds.

Megan showed Sarah and Luke how to help Janie engage Finn with finger plays, songs, and by handing him toys. Sarah and Luke continued to play movement-centered games with Janie, like dancing, dress-up, and obstacle courses. The kids also modeled using people's names when making a request. As with previous family sessions, Sarah and Luke carried what they learned from Megan into their everyday lives with Janie.

Six Months of Speech Therapy

Abby noted in March that Janie regularly verbalized her preferences. For example, Janie would say, "I want xylophone," and "Abby sing frog." "Thank you" came out a bit as well. Although her spontaneous requests became more frequent, Abby often prompted her with, "Tell me." Janie sometimes needed cueing with "Yes or no?" to answer a question. Abby encouraged us to instead say the "y" or "n" sound to help fade out that cue.

Janie's spontaneous sentences were increasing in speech sessions, such as "I get the pink ball," and "That a crab." Her vocabulary was growing, and she consistently labeled on demand (named an indicated picture or object). Abby noted that "Janie often used 'you' instead of 'I' when referring to herself." They also worked on discriminating pronouns.

Ann Marie joined Abby one session for a six-month

review of Janie's speech therapy. She recorded their primary speech goal for Janie: "We want Janie to use language more spontaneously and rely less on learned, scripted language so that she can communicate more naturally with others."

Talking about Janie's Diagnosis

I volunteered in Sarah's third grade classroom one day in the spring. On the way out, I ran into the coordinator of our town's integrated preschool, and we spoke briefly. As I walked to my car, another mother asked how I knew the preschool coordinator. I explained that my two-year-old was on the autism spectrum, so she would attend the integrated preschool in the fall.

"My son went there," she said. "He has PDD-NOS, but it's not something we usually share with other people."

"That's what Janie has," I said, realizing how much louder my voice was than hers. She went on to tell me about their preschool experience, but I could not focus on her words beyond the fact that she rarely disclosed her child's diagnosis. Her son was in third grade. I had not thought ahead to third grade.

I didn't broadcast Janie's diagnosis, but I did not hide it either. Two girls from Janie's ballet class planned to go to the integrated preschool as "typical" kids (children who do not need special education services). To those mothers, I did mention that Janie had autism. They both said they had no idea, and I have no idea if this was true or not. I am sure they noticed Janie often in her own world during the class, but the connection to autism is not always obvious.

I never felt ashamed of or embarrassed by her diagnosis, though at that moment I realized there was more to it than my feelings. *Was I doing a disservice to Janie by telling people she was on the spectrum?*

When Megan came the next day, I asked her advice. Megan listened, then told me, "It's a personal decision. There is no right or wrong answer. It's really whatever you are comfortable with and makes sense to you. Certainly her diagnosis is not everyone's business. Janie is so young, she doesn't understand what the diagnosis means and neither do her peers. You should reevaluate as Janie gets older whom you tell and don't tell. Your decision will really depend on how she's doing. If it's not apparent that she has autism, and there aren't issues when she plays with other children, there may be no reason to tell people. But if she's playing with another child and struggling in a certain area, it may make sense to let the parent know."

When Janie is older, she can choose if and what to share about her autism. In the meantime, I began to curb what I said about her diagnosis, except with close friends and family. If the occasion comes up with someone I do not know well, I usually say she has communication and social delays and discuss her diagnosis only if the conversation leads there.

13

SOCIAL LEAPS

Our hibernation slowly came to an end as winter turned to spring, and we could venture outside a bit more. Sarah's soccer season started up, while Luke tried out golf and baseball for the first time. I took the kids on walks almost daily, pushing the little ones in a double stroller while Sarah and Luke walked with me. Janie and Finn were content observing and sleeping in the stroller. Going on a walk was usually not Sarah and Luke's first choice, so I told stories to keep them happy too.

The kids ate most of their meals at our kitchen island, and Finn often fussed if he could not see them. Once he could hold his head up, we sat him in a Bumbo seat (a soft little chair that molds around the contours of a baby's body) and perched him on the island, so that he could be with his siblings at mealtimes. He would grab anything within reach —flowers, cups, even lifting a half-full gallon of milk. By spring he could sit up himself and moved to a booster seat alongside the other kids. I loved seeing the four of them lined up at the island.

Finn and Janie were both entering more and more into the social fold of our family.

• • •

Emotions Around the Family

In tandem with her rapidly improving communication skills, Janie was also making huge gains socially within the family and community. She became more sensitive to family members' comings and goings, whereas in the past she had paid little attention. Because I learned so much watching Megan interact with Janie, I rarely missed their therapy sessions. During one session when my mother-in-law was watching the kids, Janie repeatedly referred to and asked for me, which Megan said was nice to see.

I missed another session while taking Finn to the doctor. Having a babysitter there instead of me was stressful to Janie. The first time she became upset Megan distracted her with bubbles, but when a remote control toy scared her, Janie cried inconsolably. Luke had been home sick, so came downstairs to calm her. Only after I returned did she fully stop crying. Even then, it took some time for me to settle her.

When we drove Sarah to a friend's house one day that winter, Janie burst into tears in her car seat. During the next few weeks, she cried for Sarah or Luke every time I dropped one of them off somewhere. Janie did not have the receptive language skills to understand that her brother and sister would return. We ended up prepping her before each drop-off, and they never left the car without saying, "Good-bye, Janie! I'll see you soon!" Though I did not like seeing Janie upset, I was heartened by her attachment to the family.

As much as she hated to part company with the rest of us, Janie still had little interest in Finn. She memorized and repeated our comments about him, saying "He's so cute," or "Finn sleeping." She patted him, kissed him, and tickled his toes as she had seen us do, but in general she was not jealous, angry, happy, or sad to be around Finn—she was indifferent toward him.

The first time I saw her show concern for Finn was when he was sick with a cold. Christopher was using a bulb syringe to clear his nose. As Finn lay on the bed getting de-clogged,

Janie knelt over him howling at Christopher, "All done! All done!"

One rainy night I took Janie and Finn to a sandwich shop to pick up dinner. I carried Finn in the bucket car seat, and Janie held my hand. On the way out, I put Finn's car seat just inside the shop's glass door so that he would not get wet while I loaded dinner and Janie into the car.

Janie cried so hysterically I could hardly buckle her into the seat. I tried to soothe her, but could not figure out why she was crying. She was looking over my shoulder, reaching toward the store, and finally yelled, "Baby Finn! Baby Finn!"

I stood in the rain, shocked at her reaction. When her screams finally knocked me back to my senses, I ran over and scooped up her brother. Once he was secure in the car, she calmed down. On the way home, I sounded like a wind-up toy saying, "You didn't want me to forget Finn! You do love him! You do love him!"

When I put her in the crib that night, instead of our pressure fix routine pushing stuffed animals on her arms, belly, and legs, I held Finn above her and pressed his feet onto her body. She laughed and signed for more.

When I gently laid Finn on her for a hug, she pushed him off and gave me an angry look. A hug was out, but at least she didn't want her brother abandoned at a sandwich shop. Good enough for me.

Early Intervention Playgroup

Janie started engaging more with people outside of the family, particularly children. Ann Marie recommended early on that Janie join a playgroup at the EI center to better prepare her for preschool. The weekly two-hour playgroup would help her understand the routine of preschool, cope with separation from me, and provide social interaction with her peers and unfamiliar adults. Hopefully she could begin to form relationships with children her own age. By the end of February, the time had arrived.

We met Megan at the EI office and brought Janie downstairs to a cavernous basement they called the "motor room," filled with rocking horses, playhouses, tunnels, ball pits, ride-on toys, a small trampoline, a swing, and other large toys. Janie beelined to the horses, and Megan joined her. I parked Finn, asleep in his bucket seat, off to the side.

Ann Marie introduced me to the two Early Intervention therapists who ran the group, Kim and Emily. I sat down with Kim to fill out a document detailing the goals of Janie's playgroup experience. She explained that their activities would revolve around a predictable routine. Megan and I would attend playgroup too, and over the next several weeks, Janie would gradually separate first from me and later from Megan. The group would consist of no more than six children, to encourage sharing and interaction with peers. We agreed that the goals would be met when Janie successfully separated from me, followed the routines of playgroup, and showed more interest in the other children.

The kids spent about 45 minutes in the playroom with their parents watching. Kim and Emily showed each child a picture of the classroom shortly before we all headed upstairs, where the mothers typically said good-bye (although Megan, Finn, and I stayed with the children). Set in the corner of the building, the classroom had two walls of windows. It was bright but also looked sparse, as the stations and toys were covered in sheets to keep the kids focused on the activity at hand.

Six tiny cube chairs faced the windows. The kids sat in these containing seats (meant to help children with sensory issues feel more enclosed and protected), said good-bye to their parents, and looked at books as they waited for a turn in the bathroom to wash their hands.

When everyone's hands were clean, they sang a hello song, addressing each of the children individually, followed by a few other songs. Kim showed them pictures of the day's activities and placed them in order on a Velcro strip along one wall. The kids then moved over to a small table to eat lunch together.

Kim and Emily's calm and patience seemed to permeate the room. They flipped over cube chairs and sat along with the kids, making comments and asking questions. One little girl could hardly sit still long enough to eat. Emily honed in on her, giving her the attention she needed to get through lunch. Megan and I kneeled next to Janie.

After lunch they moved from activity to activity with pictures a few minutes before each switch to let the kids know what would come next. The teachers pulled away a sheet to reveal an activity station or brought out big, fun toys from the closet, such as plastic zoo animals or a huge car set. Next, they moved onto a sensory activity, usually a flour, sand, or rice table filled with cups, sifters, and measuring spoons. The kids did creative, seasonal art projects each week as well, often involving finger painting, dot paints, or shaving cream.

The kids ended up back where they started in their lined-up cube seats to sing songs about fish, duckies, and choo-choo trains with accompanying stuffed animals. They finished by singing good-bye to each of the children. Then they all called out together for the moms to come in.

Janie quietly and happily participated in playgroup. Throughout March, Megan and I both attended with her. I gradually limited my involvement, often nursing Finn off to the side, where Janie came to me for hugs and reassurance every so often. Megan guided Janie through activities, sitting next to her while she ate and facilitating her interactions with other kids at the sand table or at craft time for example. Janie slowly became comfortable with these new children, not playing with them but sometimes responding to them, such as handing her neighbor a grape at lunch.

After about four weeks, we decided Janie was ready to take on playgroup without me. I joined her in the motor room, but let Megan take the lead on interacting with her. When the kids moved into the classroom, I settled Janie into her seat and gave her a quick kiss good-bye. Megan had warned me against prolonged good-byes. I took Finn into the room next door with the other mothers. A closet full of toys connected the two rooms with a two-way mirror to observe. The closet was so tiny and overflowing with toys we took turns shimmying in to watch.

Janie did fine while engaged in an activity, but asked for me during transitions and downtime. She never became so upset that I had to come in. The therapists were masters at redirection and swooped in when she looked distressed. Over the next few weeks as Janie became more comfortable with Kim and Emily, Megan hung back a bit as well, not sitting right next to her at lunch and during the activities. Janie asked for me less and less during playgroup as the weeks progressed.

I was playing with Finn one day in the waiting room when a mother came in from watching the kids through the two-way mirror, her face drawn. She told us how her son was throwing toys and not following along in any of the activities. Kelly, the occupational therapist who had evaluated Janie, was subbing in for Kim that day. When she came into the closet a short while later to grab a toy, the mother apologized for her son's behavior.

Kelly looked at the mother with her twinkling eyes and said, "He's working so hard." Then she smiled and went back into the room. I think of those words often when Janie struggles.

As the weather warmed up, motor time moved outside to the playground filled with push cars, swings, tricycles, playscapes, see-saws, and sandboxes—all well-played with but engaging toys. Megan noted Janie's progress one day in April, "Janie enjoyed gross motor play outside with peers and was copying others' actions to explore new materials. During group, she ate lunch, participated with sensory play, and artwork. She is imitating objects' use during circle time. She is beginning to show more interest in watching peers."

Megan could not attend playgroup one day in May. I thought Janie was ready to try going by herself. Megan agreed. I walked Janie up from the motor room, kissed her good-bye as she sat in the cube chair, and headed to the waiting room. She transitioned without a hitch. Granted, she had by now attended playgroup for more than two months with either Megan or both of us in tow—but engaging independently in a community group was a huge leap for her. She now had the confidence and independence to go it on her own.

In mid-June, Janie attended her last playgroup. By then she showed interest in and talked about the other children in the group, although played more parallel than with them. The last playgroup wrapped up on a sunny, warm day at the playground. I thanked Emily and Kim. Watching Janie hug them good-bye, I again felt tremendously grateful to the incredible people who had come into our lives since Janie's diagnosis to help her better understand and engage in the world around her.

14

ANXIETY

Janie's Stressors

Janie's period of regression was the first indication that she struggled with anxiety. Her stress peaked after the holidays and lingered through the winter, always more pronounced when she was sick. Her anxiety manifested most often during transitions and around unfamiliar adults.

When stressed, Janie had a low tipping point—she was easily upset and less flexible in play and in our daily routine. Her sleep would usually be off too, as she often woke up during the night. She would also become more emotional and sometimes fearful. Megan described her as having "low frustration tolerance." Janie would draw into herself and cling to me during her ballet and music classes. She pulled out her electronic toys and carried two objects more frequently as well. In response to the anxiety, she sought to regulate herself through sensory seeking behavior like running and jumping.

Transitioning from one activity to another could trigger anxiety for Janie. At the end of a bath, Janie would often spring to her feet and in a pressured voice quote a line from *Dora the Explorer*, "Up! Up! Up! Stand up!" Echoing those words expressed her tension at the change in activity.

Throughout March and April, several new adults entered

Janie's space. Teachers from the preschool she would attend in the fall came to the house to watch a few of Megan's sessions. Janie also had a speech evaluation at the preschool and another Early Intervention assessment. She sometimes covered her face with her hand to block out the sight of unfamiliar adults during these evaluations. With so many people observing her over those weeks, she was clearly affected.

During therapy sessions with Megan and Abby, Janie now wanted me close. Her attention uneven, she frequently needed redirection. Megan recommended that I check in with Janie with a hug or question when she appeared tense, but to do the best I could not to remove her from an activity or hold her for a long period of time.

Janie's stress at the doctor's office was off the charts. While she was fine at her two-year well visit, every time we had gone in since then Janie typically screamed from start to finish, even during her siblings' appointments. When I took her to the pediatric ophthalmologist for a blocked tear duct, the doctor spent about 10 seconds gently touching her face to get a look. Janie cried hysterically at such a high pitch, I could hardly hear a word he said as he politely explained that the tear duct should resolve itself.

In an effort to allay her fears, Megan lent us an *Elmo Goes to the Doctor* book. We also played with a toy doctor kit, taking turns being doctor and patient, and explained that a doctor never tries to hurt anyone.

Janie has always been bothered by loud noises. She hated our ball popper toy and remote control toys, especially remote control cars that Luke sometimes chased her with. At four, she still will not let me blow-dry her hair, and electric toothbrushes are out of the question. During one session, when a repairman was using a power drill in the living room, Megan noted, "Janie became very sad in response to the noise and had difficulty recovering from the stress of it."

As children with autism get older, more symptoms can surface, with anxiety being a common one. While I held back from asking Megan how acute she thought Janie's anxiety might be in a few years, I did relay my concern.

"You can't worry ahead of yourself," Megan told me. "Her anxiety could be a problem or she might not have any at all. But to worry about it now does no good either way."

Calming Janie's Anxiety

During a session in March, Megan reported in her note, "Janie was a bit overaroused today which was demonstrated by high activity level, decreased eye contact, and pressured speech." Megan often handled Janie's overstimulation by squeezing her arms and legs and putting pressure on her with pillows. On this particular day, Megan laid Janie on a blanket and snugly rolled her up. She sang lullabies as she rocked Janie in her arms. Janie was as serene as I've ever seen her, silent and still, her eyes peeking out over the blanket. They moved quietly onto a book. Janie was regulated the rest of the session.

Another day when Janie became upset transitioning to a new activity, Megan wrapped her up tightly and noted that she "calmed quickly...After this, she stayed with me throughout the session."

Rolling Janie in a blanket became our go-to stress release for her. We incorporated it into her bedtime routine as well. At a playdate one day, we rolled Janie up after her friend, Jack, took a toy she wanted. Jack watched and then asked his mother to roll him up too.

Megan always finished an activity by cleaning up the materials. I now understood how the clear start and end of an activity helped Janie move on to the next one.

Anxiety and the Seasons

As the weather warmed up and Janie stayed healthy, her anxiety decreased markedly. In April, she occasionally had trouble regulating, evidenced by her short attention span and louder voice. Megan handled these instances with quiet sensory routines, songs, squeezing, or wrapping Janie in a blanket before they shifted to a new activity. We continued to roll her up before bed and at times of stress, but she had less need for it as we moved into May.

Janie's anxiety was minimal by the start of summer, but still stemmed from transitions. In one session, she became upset trying to communicate the game she wanted to play with dolls. She recovered quickly when Megan redirected her. She often let Janie play on her own for a few minutes between activities to help smooth the transition.

At her three-year checkup in the middle of summer, Janie's behavior was completely unexpected. For the first time, she followed the doctor's directions and was comfortable with the doctor touching her, even chatty. The doctor, nurse, and I caught each others' eyes throughout the appointment, exchanging pleasantly shocked expressions.

The Michigan Test

As part of Janie's six-month Early Intervention review, our supervisor Ann Marie offered to do a formal evaluation of Janie in relation to other children her age by administering the Michigan Test, an early childhood assessment tool used to determine physical, cognitive, and social delays. In April, the EI team arrived again with their bags of toys.

Janie occasionally covered her face with her hands, but overall enjoyed most of the activities and interacted comfortably with the EI therapist (who was unfamiliar to her). At this point, I was thrilled with Janie's progress and the positive feedback coming from Megan, the other EI therapists, and Dr. Shaw. So getting the results of the Michigan Test was disheartening. At 32 months of age, Janie demonstrated skills at the following age levels:

Social Emotional: 22 months

Cognition: 28 months
Receptive Language: 24 months
Expressive Language: 24 months
Fine Motor: 27 months
Gross Motor: 28 months
Adaptive – Feeding: 28 months
Adaptive – Dressing: 31 months
Adaptive – Toileting: 15 months

She was four to 10 months behind in most areas. Considering she was not yet three years old, these gaps were large. When Sarah and Luke started school, I hoped they would excel academically. With Janie, I worried that she would simply make friends. In retrospect, I think how foolish I was not to appreciate that Sarah and Luke had plenty of friends and no special needs.

The Michigan Test bothered me for a few days, but then I moved on. Janie was trailblazing—the test reminded me that it was a long trail.

Danger Anxiety

Janie had no concept of danger, causing much anxiety for me. As the weather warmed up, Janie put on her running shoes. She learned to unlock the front door and bolt out. We put a latch high on the door so she could no longer open it on her own. We watched her like hawks when we played outside since she often took off. We always yelled for her to stop, but she only looked back to giggle at us, never breaking stride. Constantly vigilant, Sarah, Luke, Christopher, or I would race after and corral her back into the yard like sheepdogs.

Megan explained that running felt good on Janie's joints and was rewarding in its own right to her—she did not have a good reason to stop. One day when Luke was catching frogs by the pond in our backyard, he saw Janie start running. As I debated grabbing shoes or going after her barefoot, Luke immediately dropped his net, leapt the fence, and chased her down.

When my father visited that spring, the kids were all running around the house playing chase. On one loop I noticed Janie no longer with them. None of us could find her inside or outside. Janie is a creature of routine, so if not running around the house to ring the front doorbell, she takes off down the stone path encircling our neighborhood. The path leads right to entrance of our cul-de-sac, along a busy street. It was one of the few times that I truly feared for Janie's safety.

I handed Finn to my dad and yelled for Sarah and Luke to look for Janie on the path. I sprinted towards the entrance of our neighborhood and turned down the path, finding her just a few yards from the street. I scooped her up tight, my heart pounding in my chest. When I returned to the house, my father was practically shaking and told me I should get a GPS device to put on Janie.

Megan increased their stop/go activities to prevent the running, though it had little effect. I also took pictures of our swing set, the stroller, and path. On Megan's advice I tried to get Janie into a habit of showing me the pictures to indicate what she wanted to do, instead of opening the door or running away. I was not consistent enough with the pictures to be effective, so we always kept close tabs on her. I also put a gate on our deck to let her be outside without access to the yard.

That spring, I bought Janie a big play car like the one the *Flintstones* drive, with her feet as the engine. The first time she climbed in, she headed straight for the busy road outside our cul-de-sac to drive alongside the other cars. If she had not loved that car so much, I would have thrown it in the trash.

Guilt Anxiety

Now and again watching Janie in therapy with Megan,

my mind would wander into guilty territory. I thought about how similar Janie was to Sarah as a toddler. Sarah was also withdrawn and reticent around new people, an observer more than a participant in her classes. Being my first child, Sarah had 100 percent of my attention. We did everything together. As number three, Janie had much less of my time early on. Even Ann Marie had told me at Janie's first EI evaluation to engage with her more. I often asked myself: *If I had focused more on Janie from day one, would she still have autism?*

I told Megan about my guilty feelings one day, not so much for reassurance, but to see if she thought that more engagement early on could have prevented her autism. As I choked out the words, I realized how heavily the thoughts weighed on me. She asked if Sarah had a speech delay when she was younger. I shook my head no.

"Sarah was reserved like Janie, but she was never on the spectrum. Your engaging Janie more would not have prevented her from having autism."

I knew Megan was right. Her words did not completely wipe away my guilt though. *If I had engaged Janie more from the start, would her autism have been less pronounced?*

I think yes. Had I known, I would have. But I didn't. And I am now. I do feel guilt over it, but I cannot wallow in that guilt. It is unproductive and, in a sense, narcissistic. It is what it is.

15

FOOD THERAPY

Janie's food therapy started with milk. I am embarrassed to admit that she still took a bottle at two and a half. She refused to drink milk any other way, so I gave her a bottle when she woke up in the morning and before bedtime. She accepted only water from a cup. Aside from kicking the bottle habit, Janie also needed to loosen her rigidity around drinking and eating in general.

Megan explained that a new food typically has to be presented to a reticent eater a number of times before they taste it, if at all. So we started by offering Janie milk in an open cup at mealtimes a few days in a row. No go; Janie would not touch it. Over the next several days, we gave her milk in a sippy cup, then in a sippy cup with a straw. No and no. By that point I was ready to throw in the towel, but Megan was not.

Finding a way to get Janie to drink milk from a cup was no different from the myriad solutions she tested out to help Janie reach other goals. On Megan's instructions, I next served up milk in an open cup with a straw. Janie drank it on the first try. I was stunned. We soon phased out the bottle, and within a few months Janie no longer cared how she took her milk.

At two, Janie was a great eater, usually happy with whatever the rest of us ate at mealtimes. The one food she did not like was fruit, so we started putting some on her plate at lunch. Janie always refused it. Megan encouraged me to let Janie move the fruit off the plate herself (so that she would become comfortable touching new foods). We also smelled fruit together, in addition to other non-food items such as flowers, to prevent her from associating smelling solely with undesirable foods.

As the months passed, Janie became rigid about other foods beyond fruit. Eventually she wouldn't try anything she had not eaten before. When we took a month-long hiatus from pancakes, she would not take a bite the next time I cooked them. It took three pancake breakfasts over a few weeks to get her back on board.

Megan often packed a small lunch and ate with Janie, pushing her to try new foods together. To counter her rigidity, we presented food in a variety of ways, so she would not fixate on how something should be served. For example, she ate cheese shredded, cubed, sliced, or cut into a funny shape. Megan encouraged dipping (such as ketchup for burgers and fries, ranch dressing for vegetables, and peanut butter for pretzels).

We also combined foods (melting cheese on toast, for example). Foods she did not like, we made more enticing—a smiley face of apples and watermelons served with umbrella toothpicks, for instance. Everyone in the family modeled eating foods Janie would not try, telling her they were yummy.

Of all the advice Megan gave me, I was the least diligent with food therapy. Consequently, Janie made little progress. Early on, Megan recommended smoothies to get some fruit into her. The road to smoothies would be serving Janie ice cream all stirred up into a liquid form, then trying a milkshake, before jumping to a smoothie. I never made it past Janie stirring up her ice cream. Food continues to be a primary focus for Janie at age four. She only drinks milk and water (she refuses to even sip anything else), and her fruit intake is limited to bananas and watermelon. On the positive side, she does mix some foods and occasionally tries small bites of something new.

16

PRESCHOOL PREP

Preschool Evaluations

Janie would age out of Early Intervention once she turned three. Our local school system would then take on responsibility for her therapy. Our town has an integrated preschool for both children with special needs and typically developing kids. The classroom teachers have degrees in special education and are assisted by a number of paraprofessionals who often work one-on-one with children. A speech pathologist, behavioral therapist, and occupational therapist are also on staff. The school evaluates each child's needs and then offers a set of services within the school setting.

Megan stressed that Janie would benefit from as much school as possible, ideally five mornings a week. Selfishly, I did not want Janie in school every morning. Obviously Janie's needs would come before my own, and at this point, she had more to learn from her peers than from me or even from Megan.

While we did not expect the preschool to offer her five mornings, we hoped for three or four. We planned to fill in the gaps with community activities or possibly enroll her in an additional preschool program. Abby recommended speech therapy twice weekly at preschool, along with one or two other children so that she would learn in a more social setting.

The coordinator of the preschool came to our house in March to speak with me about the program and observe Janie in a session with Megan. While we talked, Janie played with Megan, often holding her hand in front of her face to block out the preschool coordinator. Children are usually evaluated at the preschool to determine services needed, or if a "typical" kid (with no special needs), to ensure they would be a strong role model or peer for the other children. After watching Janie for a while, the coordinator decided the evaluation should take place at our home during therapy with Megan. She figured that Janie would be too uncomfortable in a new environment to adequately assess her skills.

Two of the preschool teachers and the behavioral therapist came to our house twice over the next couple of weeks. Janie covered her face with her hand again, so they did not try to engage her. They asked all about her and were especially interested in ESDM therapy.

They introduced me to Michelle Garcia Winner's Social Thinking learning model, which much of the school's curriculum is based upon. Social Thinking is a highly effective methodology for helping children understand social situations as well as their own and others' feelings. When I look into new programs and therapists for Janie, I now only consider those that integrate Social Thinking into their approaches.

Janie's speech evaluation did take place at the preschool in the language pathologist's office. She presented Janie with a variety of toys and asked her questions. Janie was mostly silent throughout the session. I felt a pang of sadness seeing her clam up, but also knew that the less skills she demonstrated the more services would be offered.

• • •

IEP Prep

An Individualized Education Program (IEP) is put in place for a child with special needs. It details how the school district will address those needs. Disabilities that fall under the IEP umbrella include autism, developmental delays (such as speech), in addition to intellectual, sensory (hearing or vision), neurological, emotional, communication, physical, specific learning, and health impairments. Parents and educators make up an IEP team, which meets annually to lay out goals, concerns, and services for the child over the next year.

IEPs were a major topic of discussion among the mothers at the Early Intervention playgroup that spring. A few complained about the minimal services offered to their children. None of the mothers lived in my town, so I was not sure what to expect.

I again called my friend Molly for advice. She had attended an IEP meeting for her son Thomas the previous year.

"IEP meetings are negotiations," she told me. "They will propose a plan to you. If you think Janie needs more services, you'll have to push for them. Be prepared to fight for what you want for Janie. Thomas got some of the services we wanted, but I wish we'd been able to get more for him. You could hire an advocate who comes to the IEP and does your arguing for you. My friend hired one and came out of that meeting with the moon and stars."

I did not hire an advocate, but I did spend several hours prepping myself. Fortunately, I also had our EI supervisor, Ann Marie.

Ann Marie spent an hour and half with me the day before the meeting. She brought along a blank IEP document and explained every section. She told me that I would be asked about my concerns for Janie, her strengths and interests, and my vision and hopes for her over the next year. I should gather my thoughts on those questions and have clear, concise answers. She also brought up questions I might want to ask them.

I needed to decide beforehand what exactly I wanted out of the meeting. What would I be happy with and what could I live with? Ann Marie reminded me that I did not need to sign the IEP if I didn't think Janie was offered enough services. We hoped for four days of preschool with speech twice a week, but I could live with three days and speech once weekly.

Ann Marie and Megan would both attend the meeting. They could not talk for me, but could support anything I said. I wrote down and revised everything I wanted to say, then practiced delivering it. Christopher was somewhat offended when I told him to let me do the talking and speak only to back me up, but acquiesced.

First IEP Meeting

Christopher and I sat at a large rectangular table in a windowless conference room with the preschool coordinator, the speech pathologist, the behavioral therapist, one of the teachers who had observed Janie at our house, Ann Marie, and Megan. The coordinator handed out the IEP documents. Ann Marie had told me during our prep to flip towards the end of the document to see the services offered, but we jumped right in so I did not have the chance. We all introduced ourselves around the table. Then I was immediately asked my concerns for Janie.

Even though Janie had been in therapy for several months, writing out my answers to their questions helped elucidate my thoughts on her autism. My concerns were two-fold: Janie's social and communication skills. She was making inroads socially, but had limited interest in and difficulty relating to children her own age; she did not understand social situations and cues; she was anxious around unfamiliar adults; and she was overly dependent on me. As for communication skills, Janie had receptive and expressive language delays; she could not comprehend abstract concepts; and she struggled with speaking naturally.

The teacher typed everything I said into her laptop. They all listened while I spoke, sometimes nodding or repeating my words back to me to ensure they were recorded correctly. When I finished, the teacher asked about Janie's strengths. I said that she was happy, curious, eager to learn, and had a fun sense of humor. Her memory and imitation skills were particularly strong. She was also physically adventurous and willing to try new things. They next asked about her interests. I ticked off music, dancing, books, puzzles, dolls, bubbles, puppets, *Little Einsteins*, *Dora the Explorer*, and *Sesame Street*.

We moved onto my hopes and vision for Janie over the school year. I hoped that Janie would increase her communication skills, especially her expressive language, speaking more naturally and in less memorized phrases. I wanted her to pick up on body language, better understand abstract concepts, and begin to initiate conversations. I hoped preschool would strengthen her social skills, especially fostering independence, with the ability to separate from me, go to school on her own with confidence, and participate in activities without me. I hoped Janie would follow and understand the routine and rules of school, and play with other children.

"What Christopher and I want most for Janie is for her to make friends," I ended, grateful to be finished. My voice had faltered on "friends," and my eyes were filling up with tears.

The teacher thanked me, then walked us through the IEP document. To start, they would address Janie's needs with "a structured, predictable routine; sensory/movement breaks as needed; modeling for peer interactions; visual schedule as needed; visuals to augment communication; engineer the environment to elicit communication."

They laid out Janie's goals for her first year at preschool, all with "prompt fading" (a cue in a social situation on how to behave, which is eventually reduced and eliminated when the behavior becomes learned) from the teacher: participating in circle time ("greeting peers, counting peers, calendar, weather, singing songs, imitating motor movements, reading story"), "transition to teacher-directed activities and complete a clear start/finish activity/project," take turns with a peer, "participate in arrival and dismissal routines," "perform two or more actions with appropriately themed toys," and "during greeting and farewell situations, Janie will orientate to the speaker and respond with a wave, 'hello,' 'hi,' 'goodbye,' or 'bye.'"

The speech pathologist then discussed her assessment of Janie. She noted Janie's limited eye contact and how she sometimes covered her face with her hand around unfamiliar adults. She wrote in the IEP, "Weaknesses include foundational language development impacting vocabulary, concept development, grammar, syntax, and pragmatics. While Janie is demonstrating the ability to use language for some critical functions (following environmental directions, one-step directions, use a head nod/shake, requesting assistance) the variety of functional skills appear to be reduced at this time."

She set benchmarks for Janie: following two-step directions, making requests by giving the teacher a picture or sentence strip, responding to yes/no questions, using two-word phrases, and identifying actions in pictures.

We then turned to the service delivery page of the IEP.

They offered Janie five mornings of preschool and two half-hour speech therapy sessions a week. I didn't know what to say.

"See, we're not so bad," the teacher smiled. They agreed Janie needed as much social interaction with her peers as possible, but thought attending two preschools too disruptive and inconsistent for her. So they figured five days a week at the integrated preschool the best option.

I thanked them over and over again.

I could hardly pay attention to the rest of the IEP. The teacher recommended I check off the box for bus service.

When I shook my head and explained that Janie would not be comfortable taking the bus, she told me I might change my mind and to check it off anyway; it could start whenever we wanted. They gave us a quick tour of the classroom, and we were out.

I brought flowers to Ann Marie and Megan the next day.

PART IV

OUT INTO THE WORLD (JANIE FROM 3 – 4 YEARS OLD)

17

LETTING GO OF TWO

We visited family in South Carolina that spring. On the last day as we packed up the car to head to the airport, I could hear Sarah and Luke laughing in the driveway. I walked out of the garage to ask them what was so funny.

"You HAVE to watch Janie!" Luke said to me. "Do it again, Janie!"

Most of the houses in that area are built a story above ground in case of flooding. Many have long staircases leading to the front door, this one included. The stairs made the shape of a diamond running up each side to the porch.

Janie was at the bottom of the steps. She stomped her foot on the ground just like Elsa as she begins building her ice castle in the movie *Frozen*. Then Janie ran up the stairs with her arms outstretched singing, "Let it go! Let it go!"

As *Frozen*ed-out as I was by that point, I asked Janie for a few encores and watched along with Sarah and Luke. Over the past several months of therapy, Janie truly had let it go—and not only her imagination. I felt emotional watching her at that moment because she had let go of so many of her symptoms of autism, embracing the world around her.

. . .

ESDM Progress

Janie's talking continued to gain momentum through the spring and summer. Although still a bit inconsistent, she responded to social greetings with eye contact, waving, and usually "Hi" to Megan when she arrived. Janie often spoke in five- to six-word rote (or memorized) phrases. Her own sentences were becoming longer, more spontaneous, and less practiced. She commented more and continued to narrate her day: "I popped big bubble," for example. Janie added to her wheelhouse phrases that begin with, "I want," "I need," and "I see." She started to ask questions, such as "What is missing?" during puzzle play. She also used people's names to make requests.

Some of her spontaneous comments were: "Oh, it's an oval!" and "I'm fixing it!" Megan noted during one summer session, "She has longer sentence structures and more novel sentence vocabulary, including comments and requests. She is using '–ing' words to describe actions."

Janie continued to push forward socially as well. She often shared joint attention by showing people objects when prompted. She followed a play partner in chase, took turns with action toys, and combined play themes with dolls. She also demonstrated conventional actions on herself, such as brushing her hair, dressing up, and looking at herself in the mirror.

In terms of fine and gross motor skills, Janie could imitate Megan's actions on Play-Doh and with markers, as well as string beads. She could also kick, throw, and roll a ball, and jump over an object.

By June, Janie had reached level three of ESDM therapy. So Megan had a new set of goals for the summer.

Summer Goals and Therapy

On the communication spectrum, we honed in on several areas over the summer. We pushed Janie to say, "I don't know" in the correct context, comment on locations (in/on/under/behind/next to/top/bottom/up/down), address people by name more frequently (such as, "Megan, I need..."), and deliver messages (for example, "Go tell Mommy you are ready for lunch."). Megan wanted Janie to more consistently respond to yes/no questions with eye contact, follow multi-step directions, and answer who, what, and where questions.

Janie identified actions in pictures and demonstrated those actions, such as throwing a ball. After reading a book together, Janie would answer Megan's questions about the story. She had played many rounds of "Hullabaloo" by that point and followed one- and two-step directions well. Megan encouraged Janie to respond appropriately to requests, such as "trade," "pass," and "share." Cognitively, Janie could sort objects into groups and use her memory to find hidden toys.

On the social side, emotions became a main focus, specifically helping Janie identify them (happy, sad, mad, and scared facial expressions, for example) with people or in pictures and to make those expressions herself. They also continued to work on turn-taking so that Janie could, as Megan put it, "share control of play."

Pretend play was still a mainstay of therapy. Megan and Janie played with *Polly Pockets*, baby dolls (with bathing, walking, and feeding sequences, as well as new scenarios, such as shopping for groceries), the toy kitchen, and rocking horses. They added toy animals and *My Little Ponies* into their block construction play and novel themes, like having a party. Janie one day spontaneously added in a greeting, "Hello panda." During another session Megan noted, "We pretended the dinosaur was 'scary,' and she was actively pretending."

Over the spring and summer, they often dressed up in front of the mirror, working on affect sharing and identifying emotions, as well as location words (under/over/on/in) and pronouns (I/you/me/mine/yours), which still confused her, although she began to correct herself.

During a Play-Doh activity one day, Janie wanted to repeat a sequence from the previous session. Megan would accommodate these requests to a point, but did not want Janie to get stuck in repetitive routines. So she varied the sequence, which Janie tolerated well.

In terms of Janie's fine motor skills, they traced letters and drew circles, crosses, squares, and diagonal lines. They completed puzzle after puzzle, particularly a large Elmo puzzle; Megan would put several pieces together and then let Janie finish it. From a gross motor standpoint, Megan wanted to make sure that Janie could hop on one foot, pedal a tricycle, throw underhand at a target, and jump forward. They often played with our collapsible tunnel, kicking and rolling balls through while incorporating directions into their play. With balls, they also worked on pronouns and location. Additionally, Megan wanted Janie to be able to dress herself and wash her hands on her own.

Everyone in the family worked on the goals with Janie. We modeled names and requests ("Janie look!" and "May I have some milk, Dad?" for example). We also stressed waving, saying "hi" and "bye," and using pronouns and location words. We tasked her with passing along messages, talked to her about feelings, played games taking turns, traced shapes, colored, tossed bean bags, played with Play-Doh, and constructed with blocks. We asked her to brush her hair, carry an item in from the car, help clear the table, and put her clothes in the hamper.

Overall during those summer months, we focused with Janie on shared control and turn-taking, trying new foods, using names, expanding her vocabulary, asking questions, following directions, and modeling conversation. Megan also outfitted Janie in a backpack in preparation for school.

Janie and Other People

Janie was surrounded by cousins during our trip to South

Carolina, including two her age who were excellent role models in terms of their communication skills, vivacity, and ability to engage her in play. This trip pushed Janie to a new level in relating to kids her age. The three girls traveled in a pack—playing dolls, building sandcastles, and pretending to be mermaids in the pool.

Janie also started copying Sarah and Luke with their friends. At Luke's birthday party that spring, the kids went wild at an indoor playspace. Right in the thick of it, Janie swung from ropes, jumped on trampolines, and climbed walls along with the big kids.

At the beach one day over the summer, Janie was so excited playing in the surf with Sarah and Luke that she ran up to complete strangers and squealed, "I jumped in the water!"

The couple laughed and said, "That's wonderful!"

I had never seen her talk to someone she didn't know, especially to share an experience. I realized then that she had not covered her face around unfamiliar adults in weeks. And she hasn't since.

Despicable Me

In late June, Megan noted, "Janie was interested and engaged, but there was more jargon [unintelligible language] and echolalia today." Both were infrequent at that point, so we were surprised to see those behaviors resurface. Megan had a joint session with Abby the next day. Janie's nonsense words and echolalia were again evident, and she often pulled in her top lip while she spoke.

Several days later, Janie was jargoning as she chased her siblings around the house. Sarah suddenly stopped in her tracks and hollered, "Janie's being a minion!" The kids recently bought a game for the iPad based on the *Despicable Me* movies, where tiny yellow creatures speak in a strange language. Janie was mimicking their speech and facial expressions. We deleted the game off all our devices and banned the movies in our house.

When Janie jargoned, Megan advised giving her words, redirecting her, and saying, "I don't understand" or "Do you want...?" all of which usually prompted more meaningful words. Unfortunately the minion talk lasted through the summer and even into the fall when she started school. More than six months passed before it finally disappeared.

Speech Therapy

In the beginning of the summer, Abby noted that Janie's vocabulary had increased significantly. She sang complete songs along with Abby on the xylophone. She used "I want" and "I need" statements appropriately. "Help" had transitioned to "I need help," for example. Abby noticed that "yes" was becoming consistent, but that Janie sometimes said "yes" when she did not understand the question. In tandem with Megan, Abby also worked with Janie on identifying basic emotions from facial expressions.

Janie could label familiar actions, such as "She blowing bubbles." With less familiar actions, she would say "doing" (for instance, "He's doing a swing."). Abby concentrated on action verbs with Janie, so that by the end of July, she used the correct verbs more often than not. Janie typically responded to locative questions like "Where is the boy?" by pointing at the boy in the book and saying, "He's right there," instead of "He's in the park." She usually needed prompts like "He's in the..." or "He's on the..." to elicit the correct answer. When asked to match sentences to pictures, Janie did well.

Abby also noticed that Janie more frequently called people by name and asked questions, such as "What's that called?" In one session, Janie initiated a pretend sequence on her own, taking the lid off a bin of toy bugs and saying, "They want to eat."

We had our last session with Abby the day before Janie turned three. Abby wrote in her final note, "Janie has made excellent progress with her speech and language skills! She is expressing her needs/wants clearly and consistently. Janie is also making appropriate comments using phrases/short sentences. She has begun to ask questions. Janie is able to respond to what, what doing, simple who questions, and is working on responses to where questions. Janie's eye contact has improved drastically, and she is sharing attention nicely. Her vocabulary continues to grow. Janie will benefit from continued vocabulary expansion to increase concept knowledge. Janie will also benefit from continued work on responses to questions."

Janie enjoyed her sessions with Abby, always beelining for her little chair when Abby arrived. Abby kept Janie's attention throughout each session, as well Sarah and Luke's, who usually sat rapt on the couch watching. I would have liked more suggestions on what I could do with Janie to help her speech along, but I often copied what I saw in their sessions and appreciated Abby's focus on reaching Janie's goals. I also liked how Abby genuinely seemed to get a kick out of my daughter, often turning her head to the side to giggle while they worked.

Wrapping Up Early Intervention

Janie aged out of Early Intervention on her third birthday in the middle of the summer. EI had surrounded us with an incredible team who guided us through Janie's first year of therapy. During Ann Marie's last official visit, I expressed to her my anxiety around leaving EI and sending Janie off into the school system with a new set of teachers and therapists.

Ann Marie said to me, "Oh you'll be happy not to have us knocking at your door anymore." I never minded them at my door. If anything, I was overwhelmingly grateful. Janie's therapy did dominate our lives that year, so there was something to be said for having intensive therapy wind down.

Of course, we could not let go of Megan. She would continue to work with Janie twice a week for hourly sessions. Once Janie aged out of EI, we paid for therapy on our own and through insurance. With Megan, we had a standard co-pay for each session. Because Janie had the PDD-NOS diagnosis, the integrated preschool was tuition-free.

A Month Without Therapy

The first half of the summer was filled with therapy for Janie and the pleasure of having her older siblings around much more often. Luke spent hours catching frogs in our pond out back, and he usually found a small one for Janie. She pulled the frogs around in her wagon or pushed them in her *Flintstones* car with Finn crawling behind. We set up an easel on our deck for Sarah to paint, and Janie liked to paint alongside her. Sarah and Luke both joined the swim team at the town pool and played tennis. The four kids had plenty of time together, which was great fun and great therapy for Janie.

We spent Janie's birthday at the beach. Sarah and Luke rode the waves with Christopher, while Janie jumped in the surf and Finn played in the sand. We flew to Colorado a few days later to visit my parents. Janie fared well the first week with all the new activities and being outdoors so much of the day. Towards the end of the trip, she became more easily upset and emotional. By the time we came home, she cried at situations that seldom bothered her before, and she often refused certain activities like changing her clothes or taking a bath.

Without a schedule or set routine she rebelled against transitions, struggling to find some element of control over our unpredictable summer days. Fortunately, the first day of school was just a week away.

18

THE THERAPY OF PRESCHOOL

First Day

We talked often about school over the summer months. Janie was excited and curious. The preschool held an open house the afternoon prior to the first day for the kids to see the classrooms and meet their teachers. Janie's teacher, Mrs. Sikes, suggested we come in the week before as well, so that Janie would have extra time to explore the class on her own.

The classroom was bright with sunshine, toys, books, and colorful letters and posters. Mrs. Sikes had a soft, Irish look to her with pale blue eyes and long, curly, dark-blond hair. She bent down to Janie's level to welcome her before they walked around the classroom together.

Finn kept to his stroller, while Sarah and Luke inspected the classroom with Janie. They played together in the toy kitchen area and out on the playground. An EI therapist had recommended spending time on the school's playground—the more familiar the better.

Sarah and Luke started up fourth and second grades a few days before Janie began preschool. I was sad to see them get on the bus, marking the end of summer days together. Sarah continued to have a maturity and calmness about her. I often found myself running decisions by her when I couldn't make up my mind—whether I should sign Luke up for soccer when he was on the fence, or which shoes to wear with a dress before I went out at night. I usually took her advice. And Luke still kept me laughing. His happy, easy-going manner relaxed me when I felt stressed.

Once the kids were back in school, Christopher and I often planned one-on-one time with Sarah and Luke on weekends, since the littler ones needed so much more of our attention—such as Christopher taking Sarah to a movie or Luke and I going out for dinner together.

On Janie's first day of school I was a bundle of nerves, but she in her sundress and tiny backpack hopped right into the car and right back out when we arrived at school. We waited at the entrance with the other preschoolers, parents, and younger siblings.

When the teachers opened the doors, Janie strolled in and stood with her classmates in line. Peeking through the crowd, I watched Janie show her mermaid doll to Mrs. Sikes and then walk with the other kids down to her classroom. She never looked back.

I could barely buckle Finn into his car seat, my arms were so shaky. I felt jittery for the next two and a half hours, until we were back at the preschool waiting for the teachers to open the doors for dismissal.

Janie ran happily into my arms. Mrs. Sikes told me that she had a great first day, except when another child pulled on her braid. Janie cried for a few minutes, but Mrs. Sikes walked her around until she recovered.

She offered to send a journal home letting me know how and what Janie did each day. This journal was wonderful. It helped me draw out more information from Janie about school and kept me looped in on any issues.

The Bus

Janie burst into school each morning. She seemed to thrive

on it. I thought I would never consider putting her on the school bus—too many unfamiliars for her—but she was doing quite well. At the same time, Finn's naps were disrupted by the drive back and forth to preschool. So we decided to give the bus a go.

On Megan's suggestion, we created a picture story of the bus picking Janie up and taking her to school. When the white van pulled into our driveway that Monday morning, I couldn't tell if Janie was terrified, in shock, or completely fine. She did not say a word when I introduced her and myself to the friendly bus driver and buckled her into the five-point harness. She was the first child on the route. Janie rode away without a good-bye, a wave, or even a glance. I watched the silhouette of her little poker face in the window of the van as it turned out of our cul-de-sac and out of sight.

I picked Janie up from school that day and the next few to ease the transition, but the teacher and driver reported that she did fine, so we made it a round-trip on the bus. There were a few different bus drivers, depending on the day of the week. Janie was happy with all of them. You could have knocked me over with a feather.

The New Normal

We fell into a nice routine. Janie clambered aboard her bus soon after Sarah and Luke hopped on theirs. After she came home, we ate lunch and then had either one-on-one time together or therapy with Megan while Finn napped. Within a few weeks of school starting, Janie was less emotionally fragile and no longer objected to changing her clothes or taking a bath.

In October, I asked to observe her class from a viewing room with a two-way mirror the teachers had shown me after the IEP meeting. The preschool coordinator escorted me down the hall into the tiny room where I settled in to watch Janie.

Mrs. Sikes had assured me from the start that Janie took to preschool well, but I felt elated—and shocked—to see first-hand just how smoothly she acclimated to this new world. Janie sat with her classmates in circle time, listening to the teacher and singing along with her peers. She transitioned to a tabletop activity, smiling all the while. She worked with an assistant teacher on picking up tiny puff balls with chop-sticks, staying well after the other kids had finished to make sure she got each one. Then she joined a few children playing in the kitchen area. She was clearly comfortable and happy—and fairly independent.

Tears blurred my eyes, and I kept saying, "I can't believe it." After about 20 minutes observing the class, the preschool coordinator began shifting from foot to foot. I knew my time was up, but I could have stayed all day.

I saw Janie take a teacher's hand to head down the hall to speech therapy, which also seemed to be going well, although the speech therapist was not particularly communicative. I emailed her to find out if she could send home a notebook or an email letting me know what they did each session, so that I could work on those things at home with Janie. She was terse in her emails and sheets home ("animal sounds," "following directions"), of which I received about half a dozen throughout the year. Despite the lack of feedback from the speech pathologist, Janie's overall preschool experience far exceeded my expectations.

Our biggest challenge that fall was the beginning of the end to Janie's naps, which faded for good after the holidays. This, of course, brought more adjustments and overtired behavior. Despite this transition, the start of preschool was a huge success. The EI playgroup, speech therapy, and ESDM therapy with Megan had brought Janie to a place where she could jump right into school.

Friends

A classmate invited Janie to her birthday party at a kids gym in October. Janie ran in like she owned the place—jumping on the trampoline, swinging from ropes, and dancing. It was the same gym where she had closed her eyes when the teachers greeted her and cried hysterically if they tried to help her with a somersault or other skills. She did not follow directions for games as well as the other children, but copied what they did as best she could. I was overcome with emotion seeing her have such fun with her classmates.

I talked with the other parents while I watched. I introduced myself to one mother who said, "Oh, you're Janie's mom! Charlie kept asking me if Janie would be at the party."

"Really? He asked if Janie would be here?"

"Yes, Charlie loves Janie. He has so much fun with her at school."

I was walking on a cloud for days after that conversation. Several weeks later at a parent coffee, another two mothers told me that their kids talked often about playing with Janie. I could hardly contain myself and called Christopher to tell him the news before I made it back to the car.

Megan encouraged as many playdates as possible, so I set one up almost weekly. Unlike her siblings' friends, Janie's playmates would also be her role models, so I was a bit more selective on the friend front. She got on well with Charlie, but they parallel-played (playing on their own next to each other) more than they played together. One little girl pulled toys out of Janie's hands and controlled the play not always nicely, so she was out. That kind of behavior is not atypical for a three-year-old, but not what I wanted Janie to model.

Her favorite friend was Georgia. Georgia was sweet, well-behaved, and her imagination ran wild too, so Janie naturally adored her. Janie was a sponge with Georgia, soaking up everything her friend taught her about play and new games.

Fortunately the feeling was mutual. Her mother did warn me that Georgia could be domineering. Georgia had strong opinions, but was always gentle drawing Janie into play. Janie was, in a way, a student of play. It worked for Janie and for me.

Towards the end of the school year, I asked Mrs. Sikes if the girls would be in the same class the next fall, as Georgia was such a great role model for Janie. Mrs. Sikes told me they would, but she did have some concern that Georgia often excluded other children from their games because she wanted Janie all to herself. I tried to act concerned myself on the phone, but had a silent victory dance happening on my end —*another child was possessive of Janie!* Not a healthy dynamic, but one I still celebrated. A year earlier I worried she would not make any friends in preschool.

Holidays

That fall, Janie showed her first real interest in the holidays. In previous years she was happy to read seasonal books, dress up as Cookie Monster for Halloween, and open gifts at Christmas, but holidays in general did not seem to register with Janie as they should with a typical two-year-old. She took all the holidays as they came, but did not understand or particularly care about them.

Now the holidays fascinated Janie. Throughout October, she asked to read our Halloween books over and over, and was thrilled to go apple picking and carve pumpkins. We debated costume ideas until we decided on *Dora the Explorer* for Janie and Dora's monkey friend Boots for Finn. She confirmed with me often that those costumes were still on. The preschool invited parents to visit the classroom on Halloween.

When I walked in with Finn, Janie bolted out of her circle of friends yelling, "Mommy!" I hugged her, then brought her back to the carpet where she sang and did the hand motions to Halloween songs with her classmates. Aside from breaking ranks when I first came in, she followed along with her class well. And she loved trick-or-treating that evening.

Christmas was similar. She asked me to sing "Jingle Bells" and "Santa Claus is Coming to Town" until she had them memorized. At a Christmas party, she sat on Santa's lap showing no fear, but possibly a little shock, completely unresponsive when the photographer asked her to look at the camera. She regained her speech a few minutes after we took her off Santa's lap and jumped up and down in excitement.

ESDM Therapy

Megan was thrilled with Janie's entry into school and continued to focus on her goals during their semi-weekly, one-hour sessions. Throughout the year, Megan concentrated on Janie's flexibility in play, understanding the reciprocity of play, and taking turns.

In particular, Janie had set notions on which toys could go together. To keep Janie from becoming too rigid during play, Megan modeled different ways that toys could be combined (toy tomatoes could go into the soup pot with toy onions, for example). Usually Janie could adjust. They played countless matching games and board games together. "Pretty Pretty Princess," "Hi-Ho Cheerio," and "Sorry!" were her favorites.

Pretend play also dominated the sessions. Megan and Janie hosted many tea parties for her dolls and played often with puppets and also princesses. They constructed house after house out of blocks with figures or animals who lived there and visitors who came to play, sleep, eat, or go on outings. In December, Janie pretended to be one of the animals in the game, then changed her voice intonation to take on different characters, which typical of Janie's play, took off from there.

Megan also worked with Janie on using names when she wanted to direct play (for example, "Sarah, can you pretend to be Ariel?"). We continued to focus on Janie's listening skills. Megan suggested creating a paper stop/go traffic light to help her begin and end activities.

We met with Dr. Shaw in the fall, one year after Janie had been diagnosed with PDD-NOS. At the end of the appointment, Dr. Shaw told me she was "stunned" by Janie's progress.

Family Therapy with Finn

Family therapy centered around Finn throughout the fall and winter. Not a gentle child, Finn by this time was crawling and enamored with Janie. He grabbed Janie and her toys whenever in range. She became frustrated and often angry with her newly mobile brother. Finn was unpredictable and a constant presence—a perfect 20 pounds of therapy for his sister. As stressful as it was for her to have to deal with this little person knocking down her meticulously arranged *Polly Pockets* and manhandling her while she watched *Little Einsteins,* he was exactly what Janie needed to relax her rigidity in many areas.

To begin with, Janie did not like Finn touching her, especially unexpectedly—grabbing her by the scruff of the neck to help himself stand up, batting at her clothes to reach a toy, or falling on top of her from unsteady feet. Megan worked with Janie on tolerating his interactions, saying things like, "Oh, Finn wants to play with you. He doesn't know how to talk, so he's touching you to ask if you want to play." We also told her to touch him back.

Finn provided ample opportunities to practice sharing and taking turns. When Janie snatched a toy from Finn, we returned it to him explaining that it was his turn. We then modeled calmly asking Finn for a turn, which Janie imitated until it became natural for her.

When Finn grabbed a toy from Janie, we handed it back to her, giving Finn the same talk. We asked Janie to offer up a turn to her brother if only for a few seconds, so that she got the concept. If she refused, we repeated the request and helped her do some part of it, such as extending the toy to him. We praised Janie when she gave Finn a turn or shared to positively reinforce the behaviors.

We taught Janie ways to engage Finn in play. I would sit with Janie, and Finn with Megan (he was smitten with her), as we rolled balls back and forth. Megan encouraged Janie to sing to Finn, sometimes with finger plays too, such as "Twinkle, Twinkle Little Star." We often positioned them to play side by side or together. Finn could not get enough of therapy.

When Finn would barrel towards her princesses neatly lined up in their castle, Janie usually let out a scream, a kind of primal warning for him to keep away. He looked to me, cried, or went after her toys anyway. She sometimes hit him when he interrupted her play or threw toys in anger when he tried to join in. I admonished the hitting and told her to pick up any tossed toys. If she resisted, I helped her pick up what she had thrown.

Megan understood that Finn could at times be too frustrating or stressful for Janie and had some ideas. She recorded in her note one day, "We worked on having Janie move to higher ground if she needs space rather than her controlling the playroom." Sometimes we set up her toys on a tabletop or bed that Finn could not reach. When Janie was sick or for another reason easily stressed, Megan recommended putting away her high interest toys, such as her *Handy Manny* toolset, so that sharing would not come up as an issue.

By winter, Janie still struggled with Finn invading her space, but slowly began to tolerate him. Over time she became comfortable with him crawling all over her (eventually without even seeming to notice), chased him around once he started walking, and sometimes held his hand.

Teacher Conference

I met with Mrs. Sikes in January to go over Janie's progress. Although she often needed prompting from teachers, Janie participated in circle time and transitioned smoothly to new activities. She took turns with peers, followed the arrival and dismissal routines, played with themed toys appropriately, and greeted others with eye contact and a wave.

On the speech side, Janie was building upon what she learned with Abby. The speech therapist wrote in her progress report: "She currently makes requests, says 'I want,' independently answers 'yes' and 'no' questions...and identifies a variety of actions in pictures." Janie could also follow two-step directions, though sometimes needed them repeated.

Mrs. Sikes was pleased with the strides Janie had made during the first half of the year as well as her overall adjustment to preschool. As we wrapped up, she told me that a boy in class named Elliot waited for Janie at the end of school each day to hold her hand as they walked to the bus together. I loved it.

Potty Training

Megan did not push potty training until Janie began to show interest in the fall. We started slowly with books and an Elmo video about using the potty. Megan thought that if Janie could stay dry for two hours at a time, she was ready. If not, we would put off potty training until she could. So we kept track in a log, and after the holidays began in earnest.

Janie's preschool teachers and Megan had two different potty-training methods. At school, they recommended going straight to underwear, taking the child to the bathroom every 30 minutes until no accidents, then upping the time by 15 minutes and so on. When accidents happened, they advised repeatedly, albeit gently, revisiting the scene and explaining why we have potties. There was no way I could get Janie to the bathroom that frequently, so I went with Megan's method of tracking how often she needed the potty (every two hours) and kept her in pull-ups. Megan thought numerous accidents in the house would bring too much stress on everyone.

Janie was happy to use the bathroom and had no issues—for the first week. She was a big fan of the potty books and memorized one of them. Once the novelty of using the toilet wore off, she lost interest. I brought her to the bathroom every 90 minutes for two months, with Janie resisting or completely refusing just about every time. In the winter, she struggled with regression, particularly due to a cough she could not kick for several weeks, so potty training became increasingly difficult. Janie especially hated being interrupted while playing to go to the bathroom.

Megan suggested food reinforcers, such as Twizzlers and M&M's. Janie at the time could not understand "if/then" statements ("If you use the potty, then you can have an M&M."), so she just became angry at not getting the candy. Next Megan recommended creating a picture story about using the potty, which Sarah drew up and Janie loved to look at, but had no effect on potty training. Megan's sticker chart was fun for Janie, but she did not associate it with using the potty either. I set my iPhone to a "Boing!" alarm every 90 minutes to signal time to go to the bathroom, but she fought me on it too. Offering up five more minutes until she was ready made no difference.

Megan seemed to have an endless supply of ideas. Next came the bag of surprises. Janie would earn a token for using the potty that she could exchange for a surprise in the bag—tiny animal figures, tubby toys, or Play-Doh. She showed interest in the bag the first few times, but it did not motivate her either. Potty training became an incredible source of stress for Janie and for me. It was a colossal effort to get her to the bathroom if I could get her there at all and was often followed by tantrums and tears, no matter the positive reinforcement I gave her verbally or with prizes and treats.

Meanwhile, Janie went potty without a hitch at preschool. Using the bathroom was part of her school routine. So we tried to make it part of her routine at home—going at the same times every day and during transitions to be more predictable for her, such as right off the bus and before meals. Again, no effect. Around this time, a friend who I had not spoken with in a while called me to catch up. When she asked how I was doing, I burst into tears hardly able to speak. Dreading that fight to the bathroom at 90-minute intervals daily over the past two months wore on me.

Megan suggested shelving it for a while. She did not want further anxiety for Janie or me around potty training. But I had to get it over with, not only for my sake, but also for Janie's. She would be four in a few months, and I wanted her to catch up with her peers as much as possible.

One day as I was cajoling her to the bathroom for the umpteenth time, grasping for anything that might get her there, I said that a monkey was in her potty. She bolted out of the sunroom and was by my side in seconds, asking what the monkey was doing in there.

"Well, he says that he's stuck in there, and you need to save him by going potty." She did.

When Sarah came home from school that day, I asked her to draw a picture of a monkey in Janie's toddler potty. To Sarah's credit, it was an awesome monkey—a mix between Curious George and Julius the Monkey.

At the next 90-minute mark, I made monkey noises and asked Janie if she heard something. She dropped her princess dolls and slowly made her way to the bathroom.

"It's coming from the potty! Can you open the lid?" I asked her. "Be careful!"

She opened it and cried, "It's a monkey!"

We were home free. Soon she started asking if it was a mean monkey or a nice monkey. We quickly learned that she liked the mean monkey plotline better, particularly when the monkey claimed her potty as his house and she could never get him out.

After a few weeks her interest in the monkey waned, so Sarah drew pictures of different animals on squares of toilet paper. We would oink, moo, or neigh to get her to race to the bathroom and see what she needed to defeat next. When we ran out of animals, we moved onto sea creatures, princesses, *Wonder Pets, Little Einsteins*, anything we could think of. We also stretched out the timeframe from 90 minutes to two and eventually three hours over several months.

We planned a trip to Disney World in the spring. I worried about losing the ground we had gained in potty training. So I arrived in Florida armed with squares of toilet paper covered in Sarah's drawings. I told Janie that the toilet in our hotel room was Mickey Mouse's potty, and she seemed honored to use Cinderella's personal potty at her castle. We ended up not needing the animated toilet paper squares. Janie didn't have one accident the entire trip.

Writing this one year later, we still tell Janie that an octopus or some other creature has taken over the potty. I know she's game if she asks, "What does he say?"

Regression

A bout of regression hit Janie in February.

We had recently moved her out of the crib and into a toddler bed in Luke's room. We kept her in the crib for so long because of her inability to follow a direction like staying in bed at night. We worried about her falling down the stairs or off the bed since she was such a jumper. But now Janie had reached the point where she understood when we told her to stay in her bed as well as more about safety. Although we had to switch her to a regular mattress on the floor since she did not like the toddler bed, she loved sharing a room with Luke. He also enjoyed having her in there with him.

Janie began to have some anxiety during the February school break, when the lack of schedule and routine elicited more protests about the potty, dressing, and bathing. This lasted well into March, as did a lingering sore throat, exacerbating her stress. For the first time in her life, she regularly became sad and inconsolable, crying for 30 to 40 minute stretches—often for no apparent reason. Squeezing and rolling her in a blanket had little effect.

At preschool, Mrs. Sikes helped children get their "engine just right" (too low is Eeyore and too high is Tigger from *Winnie the Pooh*).[1] So we copied that model and sometimes sat Janie on a beanbag with a book to help draw her out of it. Mrs. Sikes' recommendation of slow breathing ("Smell the flowers, blow out the candles") and the yoga she also learned at school calmed her too.

Janie started having night terrors, suddenly waking very upset and fearful. She was unresponsive when I tried to soothe her, sometimes for more than half an hour. Also a first, Janie was reluctant to get on the school bus a few mornings. Megan felt we should keep routines as set as possible for Janie and advised me to put her on the bus even if she was crying. I was in close communication with Mrs. Sikes through her regression. Interestingly enough, Janie was completely fine at preschool. The routine and structure of school regulated her.

In addition to keeping her schedule and activities consistent, Megan suggested offering Janie choices during transitions to give her some control. To ease into a new activity, I might ask her, "Would you like to eat or take a bath first?" Sarah drew a visual sequence for daily activities so she knew what to expect each day (for example: wake up, breakfast, bus, school).

We had been to the doctor's office several times over the winter for her sore throat and cough, and in March, the pediatrician prescribed an antibiotic. Within days, the crying and her overall fragility dissipated.

Like her regression the year before, Janie came out stronger. Her communication and social skills leapt forward. I was concerned about the trip to Disney World, not only from the potty training standpoint, but also how the change in place and routine would affect her. Mrs. Sikes thought the crowds might cause her stress too. At school one day, the gym where they often played for recess was more packed than usual. Janie became upset and had to return to the classroom. Mrs. Sikes recommended picture stories to prepare her for the trip and much planning ahead, which I did do.

Christopher and I disagreed over whether to get the Disney special needs pass that would allow Janie to skip the lines. He did not want her treated differently than other children. I worried that she didn't understand the concept of waiting in line well enough to last more than 10 or 15 minutes. Plus, Janie, her siblings, Christopher, and I had all worked hard over these past two years battling her symptoms of autism. If Disney would let us cut the lines, I figured we had earned it. In the end, Disney changed the rules so that instead of waiting in line, with the special needs pass we could check in at a ride and then return in the wait time. We did do that one day, but mainly we arrived to the park early, made lots of reservations, and left at noon when the crowds swarmed.

My entire family came to Disney—eleven cousins and nine adults, so it was a crew. To my surprise, Janie loved just about every second of the trip. She delighted in her cousins, especially the two girls her own age who were just as into princesses as she. Janie was ecstatic during lunch at Cinderella's Castle. Nothing I said or did could keep Janie in her seat when each princess appeared. She darted out from the table and chatted with every one of them.

Janie enjoyed the rides too. The only time she became upset was when we could not go on Cinderella's carousel because of the long line. She did not understand why she had to wait as I had expected. Janie did ask when we were going home a few times. She loved Disney, being with her cousins and grandparents, the pool, and the beach—but she still craved the stability of home.

Second IEP Meeting

Individualized Education Programs (IEPs) are reviewed annually. I met with Mrs. Sikes, the preschool coordinator, the speech pathologist, and Megan for Janie's IEP meeting in May. Mrs. Sikes kept in such close contact with me through emails, phone calls, and the daily journal that she did not have much to add to what I already knew about Janie's school experience.

I had written out my hopes and vision for her: "I hope that next year is as great as this one has been for Janie. We hope that Janie continues to develop her social skills, make new friends, and strengthen her friendships. We hope that she'll start to have a better understanding of other people's points of view and social situations in general. We hope to lessen her rigidity and increase her ability to follow rules. We hope that she'll better understand the social cues of communication and continue to increase her ability to follow directions, understand abstract concepts, and overall understand the social use of communication."

The speech therapist, as un-loquacious as I found her throughout the school year, was the most enlightening about Janie. She had given Janie a number of language tests. At the meeting, she handed me a seven-page report on the results. Despite her progress socially, Janie's communication skills needed more attention. Her expressive language skills continued to increase steadily. (Not long after, Megan also noted that Janie was offering much fuller responses to questions, saying things like: "My swimming is at Georgia's grandmother's house.") However, her receptive language still lagged.

Although Janie's communication skills were growing, she

struggled reading body language and social cues in particular. The speech pathologist wrote, "Janie's performance indicates that she demonstrates difficulty with specific aspects of social thinking, including: thinking with her eyes, whole body listening, identifying emotions with describing pictures, capturing the overall social theme of pictures, and labeling the environmental context."

Much of what the speech therapist referred to was part of Michelle Garcia Winner's Social Thinking Methodology.[2] "Whole body listening" means using more than one's ears to focus on a speaker, such as orienting one's body toward and looking at the speaker ("thinking with your eyes") and keeping one's mouth, hands, and feet still.[3]

She reported that Janie had reached many benchmarks on her previous IEP and laid out a new set of goals for the upcoming year: using whole body listening, identifying what others might be feeling based on their body language and facial expressions, understanding a group plan, pointing to where another person is looking, following three-step directions, and answering who, what, where, and when questions.

Mrs. Sikes' goals for Janie were to better follow the rules of circle time (raising her hand, waiting her turn to speak, and listening to peers, instead of "blurting"), starting and finishing table-top activities, asking friends to play, conversing with peers, and identifying emotions in herself, others, and in pictures. Janie could already do many of these things, but not consistently and typically needed cues from teachers, often due to her limited understanding of body language.

Megan had recently played "I Spy" with Janie, where she had to follow Megan's gaze to figure out what she was looking at. I was shocked at Janie's inability to do so. When they played hide-and-seek, I would stare at Megan's hiding spot and tell Janie to find her in the place I was looking. Only after several rounds could she reliably find Megan by following my gaze. The speech pathologist worked in the same vein with Janie. Megan continued with a strong push, as did I.

Fortunately, Janie was a fan of "I Spy." We played in the car one day on the way back from Finn's first haircut. I spied a flag, which Janie found. Then she volunteered, "I spy a baby missing his curls."

After the IEP meeting, Megan suggested that Janie drop down from two to one weekly session with her and to add in speech therapy outside of school. The speech pathologist had me convinced this should be a focus going forward, but I had not considered scaling back with Megan.

A few days later, Megan sat on the floor of our sunroom with Janie, toys sprawled out around them, when we brought up the topic again. We both agreed on finding a speech therapist to augment what Janie worked on in school.

"So in the fall, I'll meet with Janie once a week," Megan said. "And we'll phase out therapy with me once she starts Kindergarten."

Megan saw my deer-in-headlights expression and quickly added, "We could still meet once a month to check-in or however often works for you once she starts elementary school. But what Janie needs most is to develop her social skills, and that will come more from her peers and school than from me."

"I thought you'd be with us until Janie leaves for college," I said, only half-joking. I never contemplated not having Megan to guide us through Janie's autism. But Megan made sense. She always did.

Early Intervention for Finn

While not common, having one child with autism does raise the odds for siblings to have the disorder as well. Dr. Shaw had mentioned the increased likelihood of autism among siblings when she diagnosed Janie. A few months after Finn turned one, I noticed that the only words he used were

"Mama," "Dada," and "Ut-oh." Our pediatrician agreed that given Janie's diagnosis we should have Early Intervention evaluate him.

I was somewhat concerned that Finn might be on the spectrum too. He did not seem to have symptoms aside from the speech delay, but Janie had very few recognizable signs of autism at his age either.

I felt a sense of déjà vu when the same Early Intervention team came to our house to assess Finn. He was 15 months old, the same age as Janie at her first EI evaluation. Unlike Janie, Finn did qualify for services at 15 months as he scored below the normal range in communication skills.

A few weeks later Finn had his own developmental therapist, Laura, who worked with him one hour a week. Finn adored Laura and usually waited by the door for her, running in excited circles when she arrived. Janie naturally settled in next to Laura while she worked with Finn, chatting away and asking to join in their activities. Laura included Janie, but I usually pulled her into the kitchen with me to play or cook together so that Laura could focus on Finn.

Over the following months I could see that Finn did not have autism. His social and communication skills filled in where they had not with Janie. He has since switched over to an EI speech therapist once a week. I am fairly confident that by the time he turns three he will no longer need speech therapy.

Interestingly, a speech delay is common among siblings of children with autism. Janie also has two cousins who had speech delays as toddlers and required Early Intervention services.

Summer School

We signed Janie up for the preschool's extended school year program over the summer. She had two open weeks between preschool ending and the start of summer school, which we filled with swim lessons, trips to the beach, visits with relatives, and playdates. She reveled in the outdoors and summertime activities. Fortunately, she now understood the danger of cars and running off—so reveled safely.

Janie was the second to be picked up and the second-to-last dropped off, so she had a 40-minute bus ride to and from school. Although I pushed for a change in route to shorten the trip, she ended up enjoying the long ride and her new friends, especially a boy who was the first pick-up and last drop-off. She usually had him laughing by the time I buckled her into the seat in the morning and when I opened the door to take her out in the afternoon.

Janie recognized all seven kids in her classroom from the school year and played often with one boy in particular. The teacher said they were chatty together (he had a speech delay), so paired them frequently during activities.

Janie went to "summer school" Monday through Thursday mornings. During those five weeks of summer school, Janie's zest for life was at full force. She rarely became upset and never cried. Although often tired, she was flexible with our daily plans. The sun was shining most days, so she played outside getting all the sensory stimulation she needed. Plus she had the routine, novelty, and excitement of school. Life was good when Janie turned four.

19

JANIE AT FOUR

Summer Unscheduled

After summer school ended, the kids and I headed to Colorado to visit my parents. Traveling alone with four kids, I was happy to witness Janie's shift into the "easy" kid category that trip. She waited patiently in security lines, used unfamiliar bathrooms, and sat quietly in her seat watching movies while I kept tabs on Finn, who antagonized the passenger in front of us when he wasn't running around the plane.

Janie swam for hours each day with a "puddle jumper" floatie (that she refused to wear the previous summer), politely colored and chatted when out to dinner, went happily with my parents whenever they took her somewhere, fished alongside us with her *Dora the Explorer* fishing rod, played with our visiting Boulder friends, and sat with her Barbies on the front of my paddleboard out on the lake. She was an angel for the first two weeks. By the third week, the wheels started to fall off.

On Megan's advice, we came up with a weekly schedule to let her know what to expect and provide some semblance of structure. I drew pictures on the schedule of one or two activities planned for each day. Janie asked to go home within the first few days of arriving. I would point to the calendar and say, "Not this week." She was fine with that initially, but by the end of the trip it was clear she yearned for home and routine.

We came back home several days before school started up again. That week was rough for Janie. She chewed everything in sight—from tiny *Polly Pocket* dresses to the t-shirts on her siblings' backs. She fought me when I asked her to use the potty or change her clothes. We often let her go to bed in whatever she wore that day to minimize the battles. All transitions between activities were a struggle. Her eating dropped off as well. She needed the structure and predictability of school.

Back to School

Janie thrived once school started up again in the fall. She immediately took to her new teacher and bus drivers. Within a few weeks, she did not mind changing clothes or being interrupted mid-activity. She played often with Georgia and made new friends in class. Janie talked about a little boy named Gus. When I met his mother at a parents' night, she had heard all about Janie too.

She also began ballet and tap lessons once a week. Dressing up in the tutu and shoes were just as fun for her as the class. I did worry about her ability to follow along consistently and distracting the teacher from the other 14 little ballerinas since I would not be in class with her this time around. I checked in with the teacher (the same one from two years ago), who waved off my concerns. I snuck a peek whenever I could. Janie pointed her toes to stretch like the other girls, sashayed across the floor, and kept up in the conga line. She got caught up staring at herself in the mirror sometimes, but otherwise was indistinguishable from her peers.

Janie, Finn, and I took a nature class together one morning a week during the fall at a local hiking area. While Finn mainly ran away from the group, Janie was all in. She caught hermit crabs and a cricket, showing them to the teacher and other kids, collected leaves, asked and answered questions, and held hands with a girl she had just met.

Janie was comfortable with new babysitters and being dropped off in the playroom at my gym. She almost always made a new friend when we went to the playground. She played with a number of different children in her class and never came home upset. She had her school groove back.

More Speech Therapy

Janie dropped down to one weekly session with Megan in January, and we added in an hour of speech therapy outside of school each week. We found a speech pathologist named Kyra who integrated Social Thinking into her sessions. Kyra kept in close contact with Megan and with Janie's speech therapist at school to ensure their goals and methods were in sync.

I had initially thought speech therapy focused solely on the pragmatics of speech, like articulation and fluency. Janie's speech therapy was fully tied into developing her social skills. Kyra helped Janie understand the nuances of communication so that she could relate better to her peers. During one session, Kyra pretended to be a classmate playing "Hungry, Hungry Hippos." Janie's job was to consider how she would approach Kyra to join in her play.

Another week, Kyra asked Janie to think of three things that she knows about her (that she likes to ski or that she has a baby, for example), then to ask her questions based on what she knows. Kyra coached her along, but Janie could do it, and we kept it up at home. In one session, Kyra gave her a piece of paper with 12 pictures on it, including scenes of the weather, stuffed animals, pets, and the beach. Then they took turns holding the "talking stick." Whoever held the talking stick picked out the subject from the sheet, while the other asked questions about it. My mother-in-law often took that sheet along when she and Janie went out to lunch together.

Kyra made a visual schedule for Janie that we referred to throughout the day. She printed and laminated about 20 simple, one-inch square images related to Janie's daily routine: lunch, dinner, school, washing her hands, and playing with Sarah and Luke, for example. There was even a picture of Megan. The images attached to a Velcro strip. Each morning we arranged the pictures together and followed the "plan" of the day. This visual schedule helped address her need for structure and predictability.

Janie's speech therapy has been integral to her progress socially. She learns concrete skills to interact with others so that she can form deeper, stronger relationships.

Sensory Stimulation

At the end of the summer, I tried to extinguish Janie's habit of chewing on anything and everything by asking her to stop or taking things out of her mouth, until Megan explained that chewing calmed and regulated Janie when she needed it. She recommended giving Janie crunchy food, like crackers or pretzel rods, or a chewy necklace to wear. She also suggested heavy work for Janie—carrying buckets of water, or to pick up her feet and let her walk on her hands like a wheelbarrow for the pressure she craved. All of these suggestions worked well.

We did our best to derail the few repetitive behaviors that appeared every so often. One day over the summer when the kids and I were swimming with friends in a small, c-shaped pool, I noticed Janie following a recurring routine. She would walk into the shallow end, swim in her floatie to the deep end, climb up the ladder, walk back to the beginning of the "c," and repeat the sequence over and over again. Fascinated by her dedication to the routine, I watched for about 15 minutes before redirecting her into play with Sarah and Luke.

On another occasion during a memory game, I had been narrating our play with comments like, "No match. Your turn!" and "You got a match! High-five!" Janie put my comments into two scripts for us to follow depending on whether or not we found a match. I said what she directed me to a few times, but when I did not respond or changed the words up, she repeated what I should say until I got it right. Megan suggested I push her to mix things up, noting that I should help her "avoid patterns of verbal rehearsal."

Janie still has a tendency to memorize songs and books (Megan had early on encouraged reading books differently each time, varying the words and talking about the pictures for just that reason). I will read a book or play a song a few times in a row for her, but redirect her to another activity if she becomes too fixated.

While music and physical activity both continue to help regulate Janie (we pull out her bouncy house often in the warmer months), books are most effective at calming her. She stacks them together in one "big" book and half recites, half makes up the words, reading to herself and her stuffed animals. When she is upset I do my best to soothe her with squeezing, breathing exercises, and finally books to help her get back to a regulated state. She often retreats to her room with her books or to play with her dolls. I always give her that time to regroup.

Rigidity

Janie still exhibits rigidity in certain areas, particularly with eating. While she refuses to try most new foods, she will mix and dip foods she knows she likes, and recently she ate her first sandwich. Overall, food will continue to be a hurdle.

She also retains some inflexibility in play. For example, she might insist that Megan be the grocer and she the customer when they play shopping. Megan responds kindly but firmly in those situations with comments like, "Well, my doll doesn't want to wear that. She's going to wear this," and move on. Janie typically pauses, then moves on too.

Behavior

Children with autism are more vulnerable to bullying than typical kids. A classmate of Sarah's, diagnosed with PDD-NOS, brought the reverse situation top of mind for me. He made comments that hurt kids' feelings, Sarah's included, but also sometimes physically hurt other children. His mother told me that he doesn't have friends because his classmates "don't get him." While I don't know him well or his specific challenges, expecting other kids to accept aggressive behavior seemed unrealistic to me. After seeing firsthand how he treated his classmates on a field trip, I felt anxious about how Janie might behave in a few years.

No child with autism is the same; each has different struggles at varying degrees of severity. As the parent of a child with mild autism, I would not be doing Janie any favors by simply blaming the diagnosis or other children for not understanding if she behaves inappropriately. In the real world of the playground, kids seek out peers they get along and have fun with—they do not want to get hurt physically or emotionally. I need to help Janie learn skills to relate with her peers and form lasting and fulfilling friendships.

That being said, I do go easier on Janie than my other kids. I hold her to the same standards as her siblings in terms of good behavior, but with more leeway and redirection. If she does not come for dinner when I call her, for instance, I give her a few minutes to ready herself for the transition. While I do not have the key to good behavior, nor am I a model parent, I do know that for Janie's social development in particular, I need to correct her inappropriate behavior, especially as she matures.

I often lean on the Social Thinking model to help Janie understand and regulate her behavior. When she becomes upset or misbehaves, I try to acknowledge her feelings: "You feel frustrated that you need to stop playing princesses to come for dinner." We also work on identifying emotions in others to help her empathize.

Following the Social Thinking curriculum, Janie's preschool teacher describes anger, frustration, sadness, and hyperactivity to the kids as "red" thoughts and feelings.[1] Red behaviors include yelling, crying, or clenching hands, for example.[2] Feeling upset, nervous, and shy are "yellow" thoughts.[3] A child is back in the "green" when calm, relaxed, and happy.[4]

The teacher identifies red feelings and behaviors to a child in the moment that he or she is feeling them. If needed, she helps the child regulate himself or herself back down to yellow and eventually green through a sensory routine or quiet activity. This way the child starts to understand and recognize their own feelings and the feelings of others. We talk about red, yellow, and green feelings at home too. When Janie is not listening or doing what I ask, I sometimes say, "I'm feeling very red right now!"

The preschool teachers also focus on "expected" and "unexpected" behaviors from the Social Thinking model.[5] Expected behaviors would include sitting quietly at circle time, whole body listening, and playing respectfully with friends and toys, for example.[6] When a child teases or laughs at a friend or grabs a toy from a playmate, the teacher might say, "That was unexpected! That gives me yellow thoughts." Then they talk about expected behavior for that specific situation. When the child acts appropriately the teacher praises them and might say, "That was expected behavior! I have happy green thoughts!"

At home I say to Janie, "You got into the tub without giving me any trouble. That was very expected behavior and makes me so glad!" Christopher gets a big kick out of the verbiage and constantly asks Janie in an overly dramatic voice, "Was that expected or unexpected?"

At four, Janie most often exhibits problem behaviors around transitions. I try to give her a five or ten minute warning that time is approaching to change activities, such as the arrival of her school bus. (An iPhone timer application that shows a slowly filling circle indicating time remaining works particularly well with Janie.) We also rely heavily on the visual schedule that Kyra made to give her a greater sense of control. I pick out the pictures of what will happen during the day, and Janie helps arrange them on the Velcro strip, sometimes adding in an activity I missed or that she would like to do. We refer to the visual schedule to see what comes next throughout the day.

Ironically, Finn has taught me much more about handling behavioral issues than Janie. At our first six-month Early Intervention check-in meeting for Finn, Ann Marie asked how I thought he was doing. I told her that his speech was coming along well with his therapist, and I no longer worried that he might have autism. What concerned me now was his behavior.

Once we cut his curls, Finn's hair straightened and turned from light brown to more blond like Luke's. They now look so alike, yet their personalities are quite different. Finn is a feisty little guy—happy, loving, and enthusiastic, but feisty. He has a fierce enthusiasm for life and a fearless nature. He will try most anything. During our food therapy sessions with Megan, he sits next to Janie and gladly finishes off anything she refuses.

Finn was for many months a biter, a hitter, and a screamer. Picking him up from the playroom at the gym, I always cringed when the babysitters told me how he had pushed or thrown toys at other children (often Janie). We set up a pack 'n' play in my room and put Finn into his "penalty box" for a few minutes whenever he misbehaved. He never complained, just stood silently leaning on the railing of the pack 'n' play with his chin resting on his arms as he served his time-out.

Walking through town one day, Finn saw another child in

a toy push car. He wanted the car and ended up sprawled out on the sidewalk throwing a full-blown tantrum in front of the post office. Passers-by stepped around him, Janie quietly held my hand, and Sarah and Luke stood over him in tears laughing. I shook my head and told the kids I was getting too old for this.

Ann Marie spent an hour and a half with me that day offering specific solutions as I relayed each problem area for Finn. She also recommended getting Finn into an Early Intervention playgroup. The EI therapist, Kim, who'd led Janie's playgroup, had openings in a parent/child group that also welcomed siblings, so Janie could come along as well.

Similar to Janie's playgroup, this one also had a predictable routine. First, the kids completed puzzles and other table top activities (such as moon sand, foam, or Play-Doh), played in the toy kitchen, searched for hidden toys in the sensory table (filled with beans or rice), or played with larger toys on the floor, like trains, cars, and building blocks.

After cleaning up the toys, Kim called everyone into a circle and sang a "hello" song mentioning each child by name, then explained what she had planned. The kids next moved to the table for an art project. Afterwards, they washed their hands and had a snack. We returned to the circle for a book and more singing, ending with the "good-bye" song, each child holding the "good-bye" hand as we sang to them individually.

Finn jumped into playgroup headfirst. He loved the variety of toys and activities, plus the anticipation of what would come next. One morning when we arrived, he ran in circles yelling, "I happy! I happy! I happy!" At clean up time, he usually sought me out and pulled me to the circle to get ready for the "hello" song. When he found a fun toy, he would yell, "Janie! Janie!" until she came to join him.

During the first couple of weeks, Finn would throw elbows trying to grab the rubber duckies Kim handed out and sometimes ripped toys out of other children's hands. Playgroup provided plenty of opportunities to address inappropriate behavior. We needed to correct him less and less as the weeks passed. At the gym, the babysitters constantly remarked on the change in Finn. I no longer had to apologize to other parents every time I worked out.

Finn will always have a fire in him. At two, he is still by far my most defiant child. But EI helped me rein in the toughest behaviors and improve his social skills dramatically, so that he can relate better to other kids.

As with any child, new behavior issues will continue to surface with Janie. I sometimes have no idea how to handle a behavioral challenge. But I do know whom to ask, and I do so often. If not a therapist, plenty of books have been written about autism and behavior. I may give Janie a few more minutes of play than her siblings before dinner, but she will eventually have to join us for the meal.

With the Family

Janie does not have favorites in the family anymore. When Christopher walks in the front door from work, she drops whatever she is playing with and runs to him screaming, "Daddy!" with her arms outstretched ready to be swept up. Sarah, who probably got more than she wished for, is Janie's go-to playmate for pretend play. Janie collapses into hysterics regularly around Luke. He is her beloved roommate and often her protector.

Janie joined me shopping the other day. I don't like to shop, so the last time the two of us went together was the day she barely uttered a word from store to store. At Barnes & Noble, Janie gave me her opinion on gifts I picked out for Sarah and Luke, pulled out toys and books she wanted herself, and agreed to settle on just one. Perched on a stool in the dressing room at J. Crew, she told me which tops looked best and asked if I needed glass slippers to go with a new dress.

As I paid, she suggested we go to a "Janie store" next. She browsed the aisles of Baby Gap commenting on what was "just beautiful" or "so fancy." She liked the dress I picked out for her and asked to try it on like I had at J. Crew. In the dressing room, she looked at herself in the mirror and said the dress was "perfect." I kept calling Christopher to tell him about it and not to expect us home anytime soon.

Finn gives Janie the most trouble—tossing balls at her, kicking over her *My Little Ponies* all arranged for a game of school, and trailing her wherever she goes, sometimes amicably, sometimes not. He is the first to throw Janie off. She has learned to recover more quickly, and to accommodate him or simply move to higher ground out of his reach if needed.

When he gets in her way more than she can tolerate, she will tell me, "Put Finn to bed." Yet she will also say, "Don't make Finn sad," if I scold him for hitting or throwing food. They are happiest dancing together or chasing one another. He entertains her without trying. Janie laughs when Finn drools into his belly button or she spots a Swedish fish he had just been eating stuck to the back of his shorts.

Janie came into my room the other night after a bad dream. When Finn woke up the next morning, I laid him next to his sleeping sister while he took a bottle. I left to brush my teeth and came back to find him holding her hand while she slept. Once he finished the bottle, he threw it aside and yelled Janie's name trying to wake her until I scooped him up.

Follow Up with Dr. Shaw

We meet with Dr. Shaw every six months to check in on Janie. She usually spends 15 to 20 minutes interacting with Janie and then asks me about her progress. At our last appointment, Dr. Shaw had little advice for us, except to keep up what we were doing. She agreed Janie would benefit from more speech therapy and also recommended plenty of playdates and socializing with peers as much as possible.

I asked Dr. Shaw how she thought Janie would do in elementary school. She did not expect Janie to need special assistance in the classroom (children can be assigned a paraeducator to help them individually in class), unless attention becomes an issue, which is not uncommon for children on the spectrum. She would most likely continue to receive speech therapy in school, but overall her elementary school experience should mainly be similar to that of a typical kid.

The difference in Janie's symptoms of autism since her diagnosis two years earlier was so marked, Dr. Shaw suggested we check in every nine months going forward.

20

THE AUTISM TREE

Autism and the Mind

After Janie's diagnosis, I often caught myself staring at her, wondering what was happening in her mind. She perceived the world so differently. Just as she struggled to understand the world around her, I wanted to understand her inner world. Autism is a part of Janie's personality and her thinking—and her mind is amazing. I want Janie to follow the beat of her own drum. I love that drum. I would never change who Janie is at her core, but I also don't want her autism to cause her to miss out on life.

Reading books by authors with autism has helped open up Janie's world to me. Although she has more severe autism than Janie, Temple Grandin has given me the deepest glimpses into Janie's mind.

Like anyone who knows anything about her, I find Grandin fascinating. She has done what people with classic autism typically could not do. That is to communicate and, even more remarkably, to communicate to the rest of the world what it is like to have autism. For decades, autism was so misunderstood it was considered a form of schizophrenia. Grandin played an integral role in demystifying autism. What she has accomplished for the autism community, as well as for more humane treatment of animals, is immeasurable.

Grandin's book *Thinking in Pictures: My Life with Autism*, was particularly enlightening for me. Her thoughts on video games, for example, related to Janie's obsession with her preschool computer toys before she started therapy.[1]

The HBO movie *Temple Grandin* portrays Grandin's experiences through her eyes and how she thinks more visually than in words. One scene poignantly captures Grandin terrified by the sound of propellers as she exits an airplane, which helped me better understand Janie's fear of the vacuum cleaner and other loud noises.[2]

I had the chance to hear Grandin speak at a college several months after Janie was diagnosed. Her talk centered on the theme of innovation and how many technological breakthroughs result from individuals focusing singularly on a solution. She observed that animals hone in on details that people tend to overlook, such as cattle stopping in a chute to avoid a streak of light. She explained that people with autism also focus on details others take no notice of, making the complexity of social signals and body language so baffling.[3]

Grandin speculated that many technology and business pioneers likely had undiagnosed autism or Asperger's Disorder. She went on to discuss how these differences add to society. She named a few quirky artists and scientists, like Vincent Van Gogh, Albert Einstein (who first spoke at three years old), Nikola Tesla, and Steve Jobs—and you had to wonder. Artists and inventors see things in new ways. The world needs people with unique perspectives.

I recently read Susan Cain's book, *Quiet: The Power of Introverts in a World that Can't Stop Talking*, based on the premise that our culture overvalues the extroverted personality and undervalues introverts.[4] Classroom desks are arranged in sets, and offices are filled with cubes so that people collaborate and work together. Cain does not deny the value of socialization and working as a team, but also considers the downsides: the group tending to follow the loudest, most persistent person instead of the most intelligent, the tendency to discourage working alone, and the resulting consequences on society. She includes powerful words from Steve Wozniak, co-founder of Apple, Inc., from his memoir *iWoz,* on the necessity of working alone for inventors and engineers.[56]

The autistic mind and the solitary personality can and do bring deep value to society. The social isolation that goes hand in hand with autism, in my opinion, should be targeted, so that people with autism can understand how to connect with others and form fulfilling personal relationships.

In memoirs I have read by writers with autism or Asperger's Disorder, they often describe intense frustration with their inability to read social contexts and cues and effectively communicate with and relate to others. Once therapy came into the picture, they felt less alone and consequently much happier, as they gained the skills to more successfully navigate social situations.

ESDM therapy draws upon Janie's interests and strengths to build her social and communication skills. The ESDM approach fosters Janie's personality, her spirit, her vivacity, while minimizing and often extinguishing the tendencies of autism that isolate and hinder her from engaging with others and developing relationships.

I do think Janie's autism gives her a fantastic inner world. She does think differently. ESDM therapy connected that inner world with the world happening around her, bringing out her creativity and imagination while giving her the skills to reduce those symptoms that closed her off from us. By bridging those two worlds, Janie can now fully engage in—and better understand—the world outside her mind.

The Autism Label

During the kids' nature class one day, another parent I became friendly with expressed concern about her daughter's sensory issues and whether she might be on the autism spectrum. I told her about Janie's therapy and that she should consider the town's integrated preschool. She held back from getting an evaluation because her mother-in-law cautioned against having her child "labeled."

In my opinion, she could not have received worse advice. I reiterated the effectiveness of Janie's therapy, how thoroughly the preschool addressed her needs, and the critical timing of helping a child with autism at an early age.

A close friend asked me recently if I initially felt reluctant to evaluate Janie because I did not want her labeled—or if possibly deep down, I simply would rather not know.

Despite the prevalence of autism and the media attention it garners, most people have limited knowledge of the disorder, and of mild autism even less so, myself included prior to Janie's diagnosis. Even the experts continue to change the defining criteria. Despite best intentions, people have preconceived notions about autism. The label "autism" or "spectrum" can cause others to come up with false conclusions about Janie and treat her differently. So I do understand why parents would not want their child prejudged by the label.

My hesitation to test Janie did not come from concern about the label or denial. I honestly thought it highly unlikely she had autism, which harkens back to misconceptions about the disorder. Several months into a pregnancy that posed risks to both the baby and me, I considered adding to our plate a seemingly unnecessary test a waste of time and emotional energy. As Janie started therapy, I began to better understand both Janie and autism—and accept the connection. Once I did, I wanted to do everything I could to help her. Right or wrong, the repercussions of the autism label were secondary to me then and remain so.

A label helps determine the services a child needs. Janie's

classmates and their parents are unaware of her diagnosis unless we tell them. Does knowing my child has autism bias teachers towards lowering their expectations for her? It is possible, but more likely they have been properly trained to address the nuanced symptoms of autism. The label helps educators better understand my child's deficits and become a part of the solution in ameliorating them.

The diagnosis gave us access to therapy and services that changed Janie's life. Early on, I asked Dr. Shaw when we would reevaluate Janie in hopes she would test off the spectrum. Now I see no reason to reevaluate her. I know the tendencies stemming from her autism better than any test could tell me at this point. And I know that she most likely would still have a diagnosis, although now it would be called Autism Spectrum Disorder, Level 1 or possibly Level 2.

To me, there is no question. Therapy soundly trumps any concerns about the label.

Therapy—The Game Changer

A few friends and relatives have asked me if I think Janie would have turned out any differently without therapy. *Wouldn't she eventually have learned to talk? Could she have worked through her symptoms on her own? Was therapy necessary?*

While impossible to quantify, I have no doubt she would be a different child without therapy. Nothing about Janie's therapy was obvious to me. I did not understand Janie's autism or know how to help her. Therapy gave us the tools to draw Janie out of her autism. I believe that many, if not most, of her symptoms of autism would have become permanent and more severe without the intervention of therapy.

To me, this is akin to questioning the necessity of physical therapy for say a torn ACL. Why not let it heal on its own? When I listened to Temple Grandin's lecture, she talked about how she used to spin around the bannister of her bed endlessly because she loved the sensation. Her mother would limit her to an hour of spinning, then made her stop and engage in the world. What if her mother had let her keep spinning?

Stars Aligned

In telling Janie's story I understand how fortunate we were on many levels. I know this is not the case for every family with a child who has autism. Our developmental pediatrician caught Janie's autism; I had no idea she was on the spectrum. And she caught it early, so Janie was diagnosed quite young, when therapy has the deepest impact. Our state offered us more therapy than we had time for, which should be, but is not the norm across the country. If Janie had been born 20, 10, or even five years earlier, she most likely would not have received the therapy she needs—or perhaps not been flagged at all.

Not every child on the spectrum has a Megan to take their hand, lead them out of their inner world, and help them understand and relate to the world around them. Not every Early Intervention supervisor is an Ann Marie. Janie's preschool recently asked me to attend a focus group on how they could improve. I honestly did not have one suggestion; they shouldn't change a thing. They provided excellent services for Janie.

Sarah and Luke have the sensitivity and gentle touch to help Janie, and Finn gave her challenges that prodded her into new territory. Understanding Janie's struggles and guiding her through them has instilled deep empathy and maturity in her older siblings that still sometimes surprise me. When they sense I am reaching the edge of my patience—for instance, when Janie refuses to stop playing with her doll house to come for a bath or when I found Finn drinking water out of the toilet with a tambourine—they swoop in with an imaginary scenario to entice Janie into the tub or a roll of paper towels to mop up. Sarah and Luke are not perfect, but they have a close relationship with each other and adore their younger siblings. They make my job easy.

Christopher held Megan's word as gospel. When I told him Megan thought our playroom too full with toys for Janie to focus, he nodded and helped unclutter it. He studies her EI notes, often as soon as he walks in the door from work. He is a great support for me and an enthusiastic therapist for Janie.

And we got lucky with Janie. ESDM therapy suited her perfectly, and she had it in her to push through many of her symptoms.

I do know the stars aligned for Janie and our family. Not everyone has access to the quality of care she has received. I know of families who moved to new towns, and even states, to get their children the therapy they need. Most people do not have the flexibility to uproot their families or leave their jobs.

No matter where they live, families with children on the spectrum or suspected of being on the spectrum, as early as possible should find a developmental pediatrician, get Early Intervention involved, and read, read, read. So much has been written on how to help children with autism. Nothing about Janie's therapy was intuitive to me, but also not rocket science. Once I understood autism and the why and how of therapy, I could help her too. Anyone can learn to be their child's therapist.

Janie's Tree

Autism is not nebulous to me anymore. When I first read about PDD-NOS, the words were mostly vague jargon to me until I recognized how the symptoms took form in my daughter. I realized that Janie didn't point because she was not attuned to other people and their body language, that she memorized as a way to understand, that her perception of the world differed vastly from mine. Autism is more concrete to me now. I can identify the symptoms and classify their branches on the autism tree—social delay, communication delay, repetitive behavior, sensory issue—and I have learned how to cut those branches back.

I may never fully understand the autism tree that grows inside of Janie. I do believe she was more in her own world before we started chopping away at her tree—a less emotional and less complicated, but detached world. She did not understand much around her, so retreated into her inner mind enveloped in autism.

When Sarah and Luke were younger, I focused on their big developmental milestones—rolling over, sitting, crawling, walking, talking. I did not fully appreciate the social milestones, like playing with their peers, that came naturally to them, but simply did not happen with Janie. So many little ticks along her developmental chart were challenges that needed to be worked on deliberately and meticulously.

The autism tree does not grow wild inside of Janie anymore. At four, Janie's biggest challenges are her need for routine and consistency, and her ability to understand social situations, body language, and other people's perspectives.

Still fuzzy to me are the branches that will grow next on Janie's tree. What new symptoms will appear? How will they manifest in Janie? We have the tools to rein in her autism, never entirely, but enough so that Janie can fully participate in the world around her—and we can be a part of her world too.

Flowers for Janie

Megan and ESDM therapy, all the amazing Early Intervention therapists, her teachers, her doctors, her peers, our family, all helped tame the branches of Janie's autism tree. There are some we continue to cut back and others that may never stop growing. The tree will always be a part of her, but will never overwhelm her again.

While Janie has come so far and put many miles behind her, the road is long. I expect we will never reach the end of that road, but the view keeps getting better the farther we go. Janie is now a child with greater social understanding and engagement. She is a happy, imaginative, and curious little girl.

A few weeks ago in the playroom at the gym, Janie saw her old friend Elliot, who used to hold hands with her while walking to the bus. He had not yet turned four, so attends preschool in the mornings this year, while Janie moved to afternoons. Seeing each other again after several months was a little like long lost love. I set up a playdate.

Elliot came over almost exactly two years after Janie first started therapy. Although a few months younger than Janie, he is at least six inches taller. His shaggy, blond hair partly covers his eyes. Two years ago, I could barely pull Janie's hair into tiny pigtails. Now her hair flows down her back into ringlets.

Janie greeted him with a wave and an enthusiastic, "Hi, Elliot! Want to play?" Elliot smiled. He whispered more than spoke and even then, very little. He followed Janie into our sunroom where she pulled out a miniature closet of dress-up shoes, and said, "Let's play princess." He stood staring.

"Elliot probably isn't into princesses," I told her.

"No," he confirmed.

"OK," she shut the toy closet and hopped to her feet. "What do you want to play?"

He was silent, so I suggested a car game, which they both took up. From there, they moved on to the collapsible tunnel and outside to the bounce house and swing set, with Finn following behind.

Janie often seems like she can hardly keep a lid on her passion for whatever she is doing or whomever she is with. Being around her is basking in that glow of happiness. I could see Elliot watching and trailing her with an unconscious smile; his eyes lit up as they played together. I am sure I had the same expression watching them.

Elliot was carrying hot pink hydrangeas when he arrived

at our house. His mother told me they went to the grocery store before coming over. In the flower aisle, Elliot said to her, "Flowers. Janie. Pink."

She deserved some flowers.

Bravo, Janie.

BIBLIOGRAPHY

Asperger, Hans. "Die Autistisehen Psychopathen im Kindesalter." *Archiv fur Psychiatrie und Nervenkrankheiten* 117 (1944): 76–136.

Autism Consortium. "How is Autism Treated?" Accessed October 14, 2012. http://www.autismconsortium.org.

Autism Consortium. "What are PDDs and ASDs?" Accessed October 14, 2012. http://www.autismconsortium.org.

Baker, Jeffrey P. "Autism at 70 – Redrawing the Boundaries." *The New England Journal of Medicine.* September 19, 2013, https://www.nejm.org/doi/10.1056/NEJMp1306380.

Blatt, Gene. "Autism developmental disorder." *Encyclopaedia Brittanica.* Last modified November 5, 2020. https://www.britannica.com/science/autism.

• • •

Cain, Susan. *Quiet: The Power of Introverts in a World that Can't Stop Talking*. New York, NY: Broadway Books, 2013.

Centers for Disease Control and Prevention (CDC). "What is 'Early Intervention'?" Last modified December 9, 2019. https://www.cdc.gov/ncbddd/actearly/parents/states.html.

Diagnostic and Statistical Manual of Mental Disorders: DSM-I. 1st edition. Arlington, VA: American Psychiatric Association, 1952.

Diagnostic and Statistical Manual of Mental Disorders: DSM-III. 3rd edition. Arlington, VA: American Psychiatric Association, 1980.

Diagnostic and Statistical Manual of Mental Disorders: DSM-III-R. 3rd edition revised. Arlington, VA: American Psychiatric Association, 1987.

Diagnostic and Statistical Manual of Mental Disorders: DSM-IV. 4th edition. Arlington, VA: American Psychiatric Association, 1994.

Diagnostic and Statistical Manual of Mental Disorders: DSM-IV-TR. 4th edition, text revision. Arlington, VA: American Psychiatric Association, 2000.

. . .

Diagnostic and Statistical Manual of Mental Disorders: DSM-5. 5th edition. Arlington, VA: American Psychiatric Association, 2013.

Grandin, Temple. "Thinking Differently: How Autism and a Visual Mind Have Shaped Temple Grandin's Life and Work." Presentation at Babson College, Wellesley, MA, February 6, 2013.

Grandin, Temple. *Thinking in Pictures: My Life with Autism.* New York, NY: Vintage Books, 2010.

Hendrix, Ryan, and Kari Zweber Palmer, Nancy Tarshis, and Michelle Garcia Winner. *We Thinkers! Series Volume 1: Social Explorers.* Santa Clara, CA: Think Social Publishing, Inc., 2013.

Hendrix, Ryan, and Kari Zweber Palmer, Nancy Tarshis, and Michelle Garcia Winner. *We Thinkers! Series Volume 2: Social Problem Solvers.* Santa Clara, CA: Think Social Publishing, Inc., 2016.

Jackson, Mick, dir. *Temple Grandin.* New York, NY: HBO Films, 2010.

Kanner, Leo. "Autistic Disturbances of Affective Contact." *Nervous Child* 2 (1943): 217-250.

• • •

Kuypers, Leah. *The Zones of Regulation: A Curriculum Designed to Foster Self-Regulation and Emotional Control.* Santa Clara, CA: Think Social Publishing, Inc., 2011.

National Institutes of Health. *Autism Spectrum Disorders: Pervasive Developmental Disorders.* Bethesda, MD: The Delano Max Wealth Institute, LLC, 2011.

National Institute of Neurological Disorders and Stroke, National Institutes of Health. "Rett Syndrome Fact Sheet." Last modified March 17, 2020. https://www.ninds.nih.gov/Disorders/Patient-Caregiver-Education/Fact-Sheets/Rett-Syndrome-Fact-Sheet.

Rogers, Sally J. and Geraldine Dawson. *Early Start Denver Model for Young Children with Autism: Promoting Language, Learning, and Engagement.* New York, NY: The Guilford Press, 2010.

Rogers, Sally J., Geraldine Dawson, and Laurie A. Vismara. *An Early Start for Your Child with Autism: Using Everyday Activities to Help Kids Connect, Communicate, and Learn.* New York, NY: The Guilford Press, 2012.

Social Thinking. "Social Thinking Methodology." Accessed November 1, 2020. https://www.socialthinking.com/social-thinking-methodology.

Vivanti, Giacomo, Ed Duncan, Geraldine Dawson, and Sally J. Rogers. *Implementing the Group-Based Early Start Denver Model for Preschoolers with Autism.* Switzerland: Springer International Publishing, AG, 2017.

Williams, Mary Sue and Sherry Shellenberger. *How Does Your Engine Run? A Leader's Guide to the Alert Program for Self-Regulation.* Albuquerque, NM: TherapyWorks, Inc., 1996.

Wozniak, Steve and Gina Smith. *iWoz: Computer Geek to Cult Icon: How I Invented the Personal Computer, Co-Founded Apple, and Had Fun Doing It.* New York, NY: W.W. Norton & Company, 2006.

NOTES

Introduction

1. Sally J. Rogers and Geraldine Dawson, *Early Start Denver Model for Young Children with Autism: Promoting Language, Learning, and Engagement* (New York, NY: The Guilford Press, 2010).

2. Clues from Toddlerhood

1. "What is 'Early Intervention'?" Centers for Disease Control and Prevention (CDC), last modified December 9, 2019, https://www.cdc.gov/ncbddd/actearly/parents/states.html.

3. Evaluation

1. Sally J. Rogers and Geraldine Dawson, *Early Start Denver Model for Young Children with Autism: Promoting Language, Learning, and Engagement* (New York, NY: The Guilford Press, 2010).

4. Diagnosis and Autism 101

1. Gene Blatt, "Autism developmental disorder," *Encyclopaedia Brittanica*, last modified November 5, 2020, https://www.britannica.com/science/autism.
2. Leo Kanner, "Autistic Disturbances of Affective Contact," *Nervous Child* 2 (1943), 249.
3. Hans Asperger, "Die Autistisehen Psychopathen im Kindesalter," *Archiv fur Psychiatrie und Nervenkrankheiten* 117 (1944), 76-136.
4. *Diagnostic and Statistical Manual of Mental Disorders* (Arlington, VA: American Psychiatric Association, 1952).
5. Jeffrey P. Baker, "Autism at 70 – Redrawing the Boundaries," *The New England Journal of Medicine* (September 19, 2013), https://www.nejm.org/doi/10.1056/NEJMp1306380.
6. *Diagnostic and Statistical Manual of Mental Disorders: DSM-III* (Arlington, VA: American Psychiatric Association, 1980).
7. *Diagnostic and Statistical Manual of Mental Disorders: DSM-III-R* (Arlington, VA: American Psychiatric Association, 1987).
8. *Diagnostic and Statistical Manual of Mental Disorders: DSM-IV* (Arlington, VA: American Psychiatric Association, 1994).

9. *Diagnostic and Statistical Manual of Mental Disorders: DSM-IV-TR* (Arlington, VA: American Psychiatric Association, 2000).
10. *Diagnostic and Statistical Manual of Mental Disorders: DSM-5* (Arlington, VA: American Psychiatric Association, 2013).
11. "What are PDDs and ASDs?" Autism Consortium, accessed October 14, 2012, http://www.autismconsortium.org.
12. Ibid.
13. Ibid.
14. Ibid.
15. Ibid.
16. Ibid.
17. National Institutes of Health, *Autism Spectrum Disorders: Pervasive Developmental Disorders* (Bethesda, MD: The Delano Max Wealth Institute, LLC, 2011).
18. Ibid.
19. *Diagnostic and Statistical Manual of Mental Disorders: DSM-IV-TR* (Arlington, VA: American Psychiatric Association, 2000).
20. Ibid.
21. "Rett Syndrome Fact Sheet," National Institute of Neurological Disorders and Stroke, National Institutes of Health, last modified March 17, 2020, https://www.ninds.nih.gov/Disorders/Patient-Caregiver-Education/Fact-Sheets/Rett-Syndrome-Fact-Sheet.
22. National Institutes of Health, *Autism Spectrum Disorders: Pervasive Developmental Disorders* (Bethesda, MD: The Delano Max Wealth Institute, LLC, 2011).
23. *Diagnostic and Statistical Manual of Mental Disorders: DSM-5* (Arlington, VA: American Psychiatric Association, 2013).
24. Ibid.
25. Ibid.
26. Ibid.
27. Ibid.
28. Ibid.
29. Ibid.
30. Ibid.
31. Ibid.
32. Ibid.
33. Ibid.
34. "What is 'Early Intervention'?" Centers for Disease Control and Prevention (CDC), last modified December 9, 2019, https://www.cdc.gov/ncbddd/actearly/parents/states.html.
35. "How is Autism Treated?" Autism Consortium, accessed October 14, 2012, http://www.autismconsortium.org.
36. Ibid.
37. National Institutes of Health, *Autism Spectrum Disorders: Pervasive Developmental Disorders* (Bethesda, MD: The Delano Max Wealth Institute, LLC, 2011).
38. "How is Autism Treated?" Autism Consortium, accessed October 14, 2012, http://www.autismconsortium.org.
39. Ibid.

40. Ibid.
41. Sally J. Rogers and Geraldine Dawson, *Early Start Denver Model for Young Children with Autism: Promoting Language, Learning, and Engagement* (New York, NY: The Guilford Press, 2010).
42. Ibid.
43. Sally J. Rogers et al., *An Early Start for Your Child with Autism: Using Everyday Activities to Help Kids Connect, Communicate, and Learn* (New York, NY: The Guilford Press, 2012).
44. Vivanti, Giacomo, et al., *Implementing the Group-Based Early Start Denver Model for Preschoolers with Autism* (Switzerland: Springer International Publishing, AG, 2017).

18. The Therapy of Preschool

1. Mary Sue Williams and Sherry Shellenberger, *How Does Your Engine Run? A Leader's Guide to the Alert Program for Self-Regulation* (Albuquerque, NM: TherapyWorks, Inc., 1996).
2. "Social Thinking Methodology," Social Thinking, accessed November 1, 2020, https://www.socialthinking.com/social-thinking-methodology.
3. Ryan Hendrix et al., *We Thinkers! Series Volume 1: Social Explorers* (Santa Clara, CA: Think Social Publishing, Inc., 2013).

19. Janie at Four

1. Leah Kuypers, *The Zones of Regulation: A Curriculum Designed to Foster Self-Regulation and Emotional Control* (Santa Clara, CA: Think Social Publishing, Inc., 2011).
2. Ibid.
3. Ibid.
4. Ibid.
5. Ryan Hendrix et al., *We Thinkers! Series Volume 2: Social Problem Solvers* (Santa Clara, CA: Think Social Publishing, 2016).
6. Ibid.

20. The Autism Tree

1. Temple Grandin, *Thinking in Pictures: My Life with Autism* (New York, NY: Vintage Books, 2010).
2. *Temple Grandin,* directed by Mick Jackson (New York, NY: HBO Films, 2010).
3. Temple Grandin, "Thinking Differently: How Autism and a Visual Mind Have Shaped Temple Grandin's Life and Work" (presentation at Babson College, Wellesley, MA, February 6, 2013).
4. Susan Cain, *Quiet: The Power of Introverts in a World that Can't Stop Talking* (New York, NY: Broadway Books, 2013).
5. Ibid.

6. Steve Wozniak and Gina Smith, *iWoz: Computer Geek to Cult Icon: How I Invented the Personal Computer, Co-Founded Apple, and Had Fun Doing It* (New York, NY: W.W. Norton & Company, 2006).